TO YOUR HEALTH

*Practical,
easy-to-understand
medical advice.*

Randal F. Wojciehoski, D.P.M., D.O. (Dr. Wojo)

dedication

To Michele, Jozef, Kasia, Mom and Dad, Nannie, Papa and Jason.

Family is the heart of wellness.

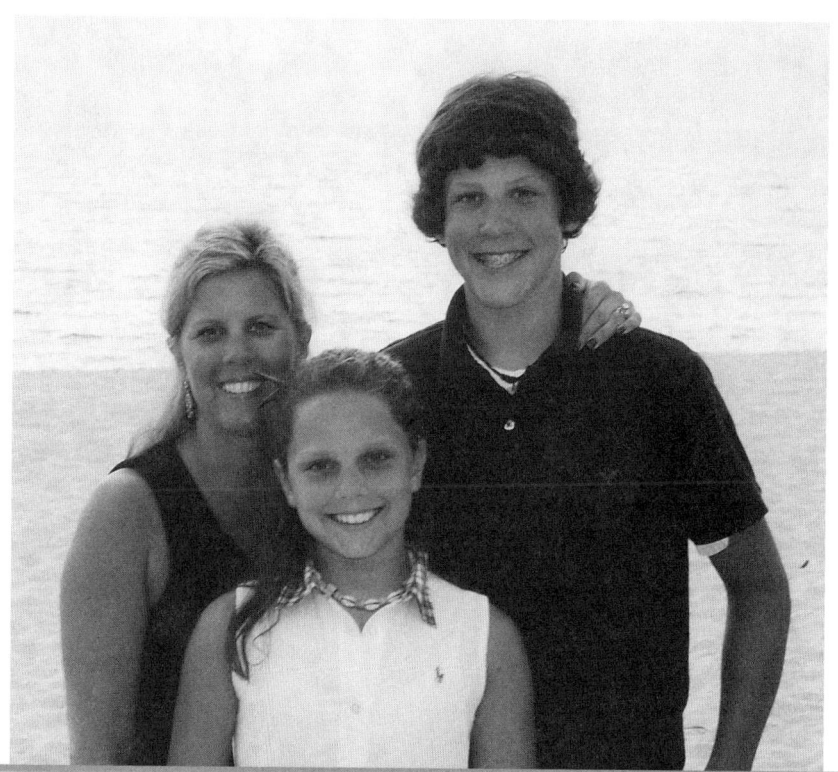

preface

As a young boy, I dreamt of becoming a doctor and having a book published. This has now come to fruition and it would not have been possible without a great deal of help from numerous individuals.

The educators in my life from Pacelli High School in Stevens Point, Wisconsin, Marquette University, The New York College of Podiatric Medicine, and the University of New College of Osteopathic Medicine all deserve credit. I was fortunate to receive outstanding training from the physicians at the Marshfield Clinic, Marshfield, Wisconsin. As a resident in a world class medical facility I was given autonomy to pursue my goals and dreams. Finally, over the past two decades, I have worked with the tremendous, dedicated physicians at St. Michael's Hospital and Ministry Health Care in Stevens Point, Wisconsin—the same hospital where I was born.

Over the years, health care has changed for both the patient and the physician. Patients have become more educated about their problems and most have the desire to learn more.
This is one reason that I began my weekly column—to serve the community by educating the community. What started for me as a community service has evolved into a syndicated medical column, "To your health, with Dr. Wojo."

Now, I have taken some of my readers' favorite topics and assembled them into this reference book of medical conditions. It is my hope that my simple advice will answer many questions and help direct the patient to appropriate medical treatment.

Above all, I am grateful to my patients and readers who have inspired me to write about their concerns. With that, I wish you all good health.

index

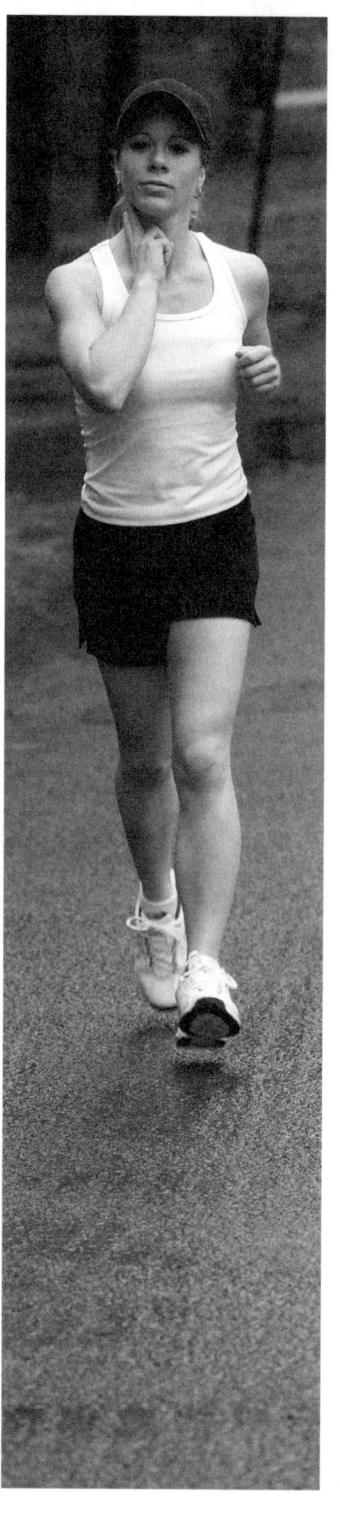

alcohol poisoning

One evening I was working in the emergency department at the local hospital, and at 3:00 a.m. I was confronted with treating three young adults in their late teens and early twenties. They were brought in at about the same time by ambulances from different locations. They had one commonality amongst them–they were all extremely intoxicated, unconscious, and vomiting.

These three very healthy young individuals all faced a life-threatening event that could have been prevented. All three of these young adults were suffering from alcohol poisoning that resulted from irresponsible drinking. Although I had to perform some invasive medical procedures to sustain life, none of these people died but the potential was there.

WHAT IS ALCOHOL POISONING? This is a serious, life-threatening medical problem that results from excessive intake of alcohol. Most commonly, alcohol poisoning results from binge drinking and college students are at greatest risk.

Alcohol is a depressant and slows body functions. Excessive intake of alcohol leads to impaired judgment and concentration. This may lead to confusion, with loss of motor function and balance. Eventually, an intoxicated individual may fall and strike his/her head. Closed head trauma may then lead to bleeding in the brain, development of seizures and permanent disability.

Alcohol is also an irritant to the stomach and excessive amounts of alcohol can lead to vomiting. This is a serious problem if you are unconscious and cannot control your airway. There are hundreds of deaths each year from people choking on their own vomitus while passed out. When patients like this come in to the hospital, it is necessary to place a tube in their airway in order to protect them from choking on their vomit. These patients are placed on a respirator until the effects of the alcohol wear off.

Several other things may happen to the body when a person suffers from alcohol poisoning. They may experience an abnormal heartbeat, which may lead to death or levels of blood sugar may be altered, leading to problems. In the Northern climates and cold, a person may pass out in the cold and suffer from hypothermia, leading to death. Alcohol actually lowers body temperature, in addition to impairing one's perception of cold weather. Most of those Packer fans with their shirts off during the December games are probably not drinking milk while at the game!

HOW COMMON IS THIS PROBLEM? This is a serious problem with our youth, and especially college students. A recent study has shown that nearly half of all college students binge drink, whereby they drink to excess once every two weeks. Unfortunately, it looks like these numbers are on the rise. It was shown that in the United States, 12 million undergraduate college students drank about 4 billion cans of beer each year. This behavior affects performance and grades in school, and sexual assaults are frequently associated with excessive drinking on our college campuses. All of these factors have tremendous implications for our health care system.

WHAT SHOULD BE DONE FOR A PATIENT WITH ALCOHOL POISONING? Most importantly, the individual must be protected from further injury. This includes protection from falls, assaults and rape. The airway must be protected and the individual must be closely watched so they do not choke. They should be placed on their side in order to help keep the airway clear of vomit. When a patient is in this state, trained medical professionals must evaluate them. This may involve calling 911 and bringing the patient to the hospital for further medical examination and treatment. Most of the time, these patients are just monitored closely for several hours. There are times when more aggressive treatment is necessary to protect an airway and sustain life.

WHAT ELSE CAN BE DONE? Sensible and legal drinking is essential. Avoid binge drinking, as this may lead to a life-long problem of alcohol-related health and legal issues. As parents, we must take an active role in the lives of our children and youth and keep them informed about the seriousness of this problem. Community awareness and education has been shown to diminish the occurrence of this life-threatening problem.

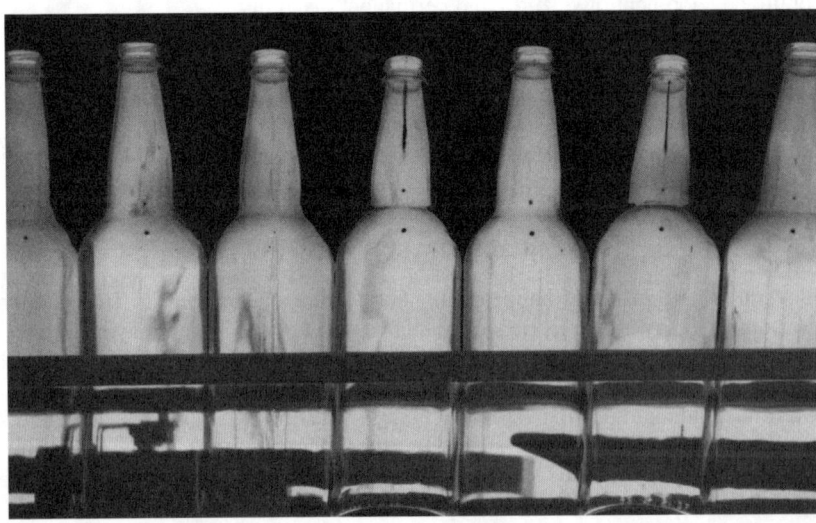

cocaine

As the holidays begin to wind down and life returns to normal, diets and overin-dulgences should stabilize as well. During the holidays, it is not uncommon to see an increase in emergency department visits for a variety of concerns such as chest pain.

Unfortunately, some cases of chest pain are self-induced due to excessive alco-hol intake or the use of cocaine. Cocaine use has been shown to be a major risk factor in the development of cardiac problems. These problems can have very serious and lifelong implications.

WHAT IS COCAINE? Cocaine is an illegal and highly-addictive drug that is an extract from the coca plant. Its use dates back over 5,000 years to South America, but reports of addiction have been cited in the United States since the early 1900s.

In the 1970s, the United States government highly regulated its medical use. At present, it is still used medically as a topical anesthetic primarily in ENT (Ear, Nose, and Throat) procedures. Due to the social and legal stigma associated with its medical use, many physicians use other anesthetics that are just as effec-tive.

HOW DOES IT WORK? Cocaine is found in many forms. Medically, it can be applied topically where it is rapidly absorbed into the body through the skin or mucous membranes, providing local anesthesia and constricting of the blood vessels in the area applied.

In terms of drug abuse, cocaine may be found in powder form and is inhaled through the nose. It may also be heated and then smoked in a form called freebasing or crack. Crack is very concentrated and the most potent form of cocaine. Drug abusers may also inject cocaine directly into their veins, which yields a very rapid absorption.

The onset of the drug varies depending on the route of administration. Inhala-tion and injection have an instantaneous onset of action, with peak effects occur-ring within an hour or two. This can have serious medical implications.

ALCOHOL/DRUGS

HOW DOES COCAINE AFFECT THE HEART? Cocaine can cause very serious damage to the heart. It is important that health care providers consider the possible use of cocaine in young patients that present with cardiac symptoms such as chest pain or heart arrhythmias.

Since cocaine causes blood vessels to constrict, cardiac vessels on the heart can be affected, interrupting the blood flow to the heart muscle. The symptoms the patient exhibits are similar to a heart attack.

It has also been shown that cocaine can cause clotting of the blood and this will also lead to the blockage of the arteries on the heart. Once again, this is the same process of a heart attack, also called a myocardial infarction.

Lastly, recent literature has also shown that cocaine can lead to atherosclerosis, which is narrowing of the arteries. In addition, the heart muscle may be damaged and enlarge the heart.

WHAT IS THE TREATMENT FOR COCAINE-INDUCED CHEST PAIN? The emergency treatment is the same for all chest pain or acute coronary syndromes. This may include the administration of aspirin, nitroglycerin and blood-thinning agents like heparin.

Beta blocking drugs are used in the treatment of acute coronary syndrome, but if a patient has been using cocaine, these drugs should not be used because they potentiate the effects of cocaine. This is very dangerous and it is important to be honest with the health care provider regarding the use of cocaine. In this instance, benzodiazepines like Valium, Versed, or Ativan will be used to calm the effects of cocaine.

Additional treatment of cocaine-induced chest pain will probably include hospitalization for cardiac monitoring. It may be necessary to undergo cardiac catheterization as well to evaluate the status of the coronary arteries.

WHAT ELSE SHOULD BE DONE? Cocaine, in all forms, is highly addictive. If you use cocaine, you must stop! Seek help from a drug treatment program. In the event that you develop cocaine-induced chest pain, seek medical attention immediately and be honest with the health care provider about your drug use, so that you will not be harmed by medications that should not be administered.

college
alcohol

Practicing in a university town means an increase in volume in the emergency department once the academic year begins. Unfortunately, each year we see a few students that have experimented with alcohol for the first time and end up, literally, on our doorstep.

Nationally, abuse of alcohol is a problem on college campuses. This may include the first-time offender, as well as the experienced drinker. Each year, several students around the country die after drinking too much.

WHAT IS ALCOHOL POISONING? This is a serious life-threatening medical problem that results from excessive intake of alcohol. Most commonly, alcohol poisoning results from binge drinking and college students are at greatest risk.

Alcohol is a depressant and slows body functions. Excessive intake of alcohol leads to impaired judgment and concentration. This may lead to confusion with loss of motor function and balance. Eventually, an intoxicated individual may fall and strike their head. Closed head trauma may lead to bleeding in the brain, development of seizures, and permanent disability.

Alcohol is also an irritant to the stomach and excessive amounts of alcohol can lead to vomiting. This is a serious problem if you are unconscious and cannot control your airway. There are hundreds of deaths each year from people choking on their own vomitus while passed out. When patients like this come in to the hospital, it is necessary to place a tube in their airway in order to protect them from choking on their vomit. These patients are placed on a respirator until the effects of the alcohol wear off.

Several other things may happen to the body when a person suffers from alcohol poisoning. They may experience an abnormal heartbeat, which may lead to death or levels of blood sugar may be altered leading to problems. In the Northern climates, a person may pass out in the cold and suffer from hypothermia leading to death. Alcohol actually lowers body temperature, in addition to impairing one's perception of cold weather. Students have been found passed out near bars and their dorms, thus suffering long-term problems from cold related-injuries.

HOW COMMON IS THIS PROBLEM? This is a serious problem with our youth, and especially college students. A recent study has shown that nearly half of all college students binge drink, whereby they drink to excess once every two weeks. Unfortunately, it looks like these numbers are on the rise. It was shown that in the United States, 12 million undergraduate college students drank about 4 billion cans of beer each year. This behavior affects performance and grades in school, and sexual assaults are frequently associated with excessive drinking on our college campuses. All of these factors have tremendous implications for our health care system.

WHAT SHOULD BE DONE FOR A PATIENT WITH ALCOHOL POISONING? Most importantly, the individual must be protected from further injury. This includes protection from falls, assaults and rape. The airway must be protected and the individual must be closely watched so they do not choke. They should be placed on their side in order to help keep the airway clear of vomit. When a patient is in this state, trained medical professionals must evaluate them. This may involve calling 911 and bringing the patient to the hospital for further medical examination and treatment. Most of the time, these patients are just monitored closely for several hours. There are times when more aggressive treatment is necessary to protect an airway and sustain life.

WHAT ELSE CAN BE DONE? As parents, prepare your children for the freedom of college life and exposure to alcohol. During the beginning of the year, keep in very close touch and assess the living situation. Sensible and legal drinking is essential. Take an active role in the lives of your children and youth and keep them informed about the seriousness of this problem. Legal and academic problems can have a life-long impact. Community awareness and education have been shown to diminish the occurrence of this avoidable problem.

ephedra

With all of the media attention directed toward athletes dying from the use of over-the-counter weight loss remedies, we have to ask ourselves if we are willing to jeopardize our lives in order to lose weight. It is time we familiarize ourselves with the common health risks associated with using weight loss products and natural medications that include the deadly ingredient, Ephedra.

WHAT IS EPHEDRA? Harvested in the fall, Ephedra comes from a shrub in Mongolia and is used for medicinal purposes. Sometimes referred to as Ma-Huang, Ephedra is associated with the drug ephedrine and it is chemically related to pseudoephedrine. Considered a natural product, Ephedra can be found in many herbal preparations.

WHAT IS EPHEDRA USED FOR? Whether in a tablet, capsule or liquid form, many natural supplements, which are not controlled by the Food and Drug Administration (FDA), contain Ephedra. Ephedra has been used for respiratory illnesses such as asthma and bronchitis, as well as to increase heart rate and blood pressure. There has been no scientific or medical evidence that supports using Ephedra to enhance weight loss. As it has been shown in the United States and in Canada, this can be a dangerous drug when used for that purpose.

WHAT ARE THE SIDE EFFECTS? The adverse side effects of Ephedra are similar to those of amphetamines, which are referred to in the general public as "speed" or "uppers." These adverse symptoms may include a headache, emotional irritability, confusion, restlessness, nausea and vomiting, insomnia, rapid heart rate, irregular heartbeats, elevated blood pressure and even stroke.

The two major concerns are the effect on the heart and blood vessels, as well as the brain. Ephedra can cause a spasm of the blood vessels and interrupt the electrical impulses in the heart. Very high doses have been known to cause hemorrhagic strokes, which are secondary to ruptured blood vessels in the brain. Heart beat irregularities and stroke were found to be the leading causes of death when linked with the use of Ephedra.

WHAT SHOULD I DO? First and foremost, it is reasonable to avoid using Ephedra. Ephedra has been found to interact with many prescription drugs such as heart medications, antidepressants and anesthetics. That is why it is very important to be honest with your doctor about the medications and supplements that you are taking. In the event that your health care provider is not aware of the supplements, a medication that could cause a serious drug interaction may be prescribed when taken in conjunction with a supplement.

If you choose to take Ephedra, do not take it when pregnant or if you have a history of heart and blood pressure problems. Do not take it if you have had a stroke or if you have glaucoma. It is also important to remember that with many medications or supplements, long-term use may lead to dependence.

WHAT ABOUT OTHER NATURAL REMEDIES? When considering the use of any natural remedy, it is very important to discuss the pros and cons with your health care provider first. There may be serious interactions with other prescribed medications you are currently taking. There has also been a lack of standardization of some herbal medicines, so quality control and dosing may be a problem. It is important to remember that just because the supplement is natural, does not automatically mean that it is safe.

Medical research has supported the use of many herbal medications, so it is very important to familiarize yourself with these studies prior to taking a natural medication or supplement such as Ephedra. As with most conditions and medications, if you have a question or concern, discuss it with your health care provider. You may be preventing the development of a permanent disability or even death!

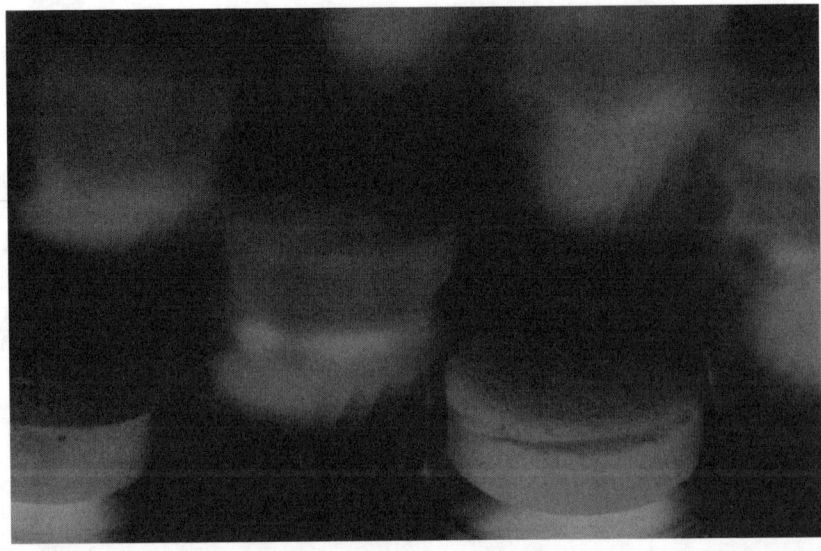

GHB Gammahydroxy-butyrate

When we prepare to send our kids off to college, there's a checklist of materials and clothes that we go over, and we also talk about credit cards, behavior and responsibility. But there is a silent wickedness out there, that both young women and men need to be warned about, because all the precautions in the world may not protect our kids from this crime.

Known on the street as "liquid X," Gammahydroxybutyrate (GHB) is circulating within the club scene and is being used for the same purpose as another street drug, Rohpnol, better knows as "Ruffies" or the "date rape" drug. Used in small doses, GHB reduces social inhibitions and increases libido. But when taken at higher doses, the euphoria gives way to feelings of sedation, and sometimes, gives way to death.

Before you talk to your kids, take a few minutes to educate yourself on this killing craze that is fooling our youth.

WHAT IS GHB? GHB is a colorless, odorless, powerful, rapid-acting central nervous system depressant. This drug was initially developed in the 1920s and was used medically in the 1960s as an anesthetic agent.

In the 1980s, health food stores sold GHB as an enhancement to body building formulas. By 1990, GHB was banned by the FDA and deemed an illegal recreational drug. At present, the drug is produced in home laboratories and sold on the street as a party drug. This drug has been implicated in several rape cases.

WHAT ARE THE EFFECTS? GHB is a nervous system relaxant and depressant. The effects are dose-dependent, meaning the larger the dose, the more intense the effects. In lower doses, the user may feel happy, euphoric and disconnected from reality. These effects are potentiated by alcohol and may lead to very severe consequences.

Higher doses may lead to dizziness, sleepiness and loss of consciousness. In very high doses, a person may be rendered completely unconscious and comatose within a few short minutes.

ALCOHOL/DRUGS

Other known side effects may include nausea, vomiting, delusions, hallucinations, low blood pressure, slow heart rate, respiratory failure and amnesia. All of the cardiovascular side effects are very, very serious. This may be coupled with unconsciousness and vomiting, which can be fatal.

HOW PREVALENT IS GHB? Several years ago, GHB was only found in big cities, but that has changed. Since 1990, there have been more than 15,000 cases of GHB use reported that have involved either an encounter with the law or a trip to the emergency room. In addition, there have been nearly one hundred deaths attributed to GHB poisoning. National studies have shown that nearly one to two percent of all high school and college students have used GHB.

IS GHB ILLEGAL? Yes. The possession, distribution, manufacture and use of GHB are illegal and can lead to a 20-year prison sentence. In addition, the use of GHB to facilitate a rape has been reported in at least 30 cases in the United States.

Unknowing victims have been given this medication, rendering them unconscious, prior to a sexual assault. Even though there have been just a few reported cases, there is the possibility that this is under-reported data. Victims may not seek help and when they do, it is impossible to test for the presence of the drug, as it is only detectable in a person's system for a very brief period.

HOW IS GHB POISONING TREATED? There is no known antidote for GHB poisoning. Usually, the most severe cases are brought to the hospital in a very critical state. The airway must be protected and the patient may not be breathing. A tube will be placed in the lungs and the patient will be placed on a respirator until the effects wear off. Respiratory efforts must be assisted until the patient is able to breathe on their own.

All of the treatment is supportive, including the use of intravenous fluids to increase blood pressure. Most of the victims of GHB poisoning will have no recollection of the events after ingestion and are usually discharged from the hospital.

WHAT ELSE SHOULD I DO? The use of GHB is very dangerous and may kill a user. The dosing is very sensitive and home labs do not yield a pure product. Do not use GHB, as one sip may render a person completely unconscious within a few minutes. If alone, a person may die from aspirating vomitus or stopped breathing.

If you witness a GHB poisoning, call 911. The patient must be evaluated and admitted for supportive therapy and observation. Studies have shown that repeated use leads to addiction. This may require drug counseling and therapy. As always, seek professional medical attention when presented with questions about drug abuse and addiction.

holiday heart

During the holiday season, we are faced with many personal and social challenges. It seems that there may be a great deal of personally-induced stress due to all of the expectations associated with the season. The emergency department is very busy during this time of the year tending to a variety of health issues related to the holidays. These conditions may include anxiety, depression, suicide, over-eating, traumatic injuries and alcohol intoxication.

In addition, there are more parties and that usually means alcohol. Many people are not used to drinking alcohol during the year, and will over-indulge. A common problem related to binge drinking during the holidays leads to some heart trouble. It has been known since 1978 that binge drinking or over indulging can lead to a heart irregularity called "holiday heart."

WHAT IS HOLIDAY HEART? This is when a person, either young or old, experiences an arrhythmia or irregular heart beat. The rate is usually very rapid and the patient will feel palpitations. This may be a sustained and isolated event and it is believed that drinking too much alcohol causes it.

It is well known that chronic alcoholism leads to numerous heart problems and damage. Alcoholics may suffer from an enlarged heart and heart failure, which is fluid on the lungs. The enlarged heart will lose its ability to pump due to the damage done to the muscle by alcohol. Cessation of drinking leads to improved cardiac function, but the effects of alcohol can be permanent.

Fortunately, with holiday heart, this is not the case. The symptoms are frightening, but will usually resolve with no permanent damage. It is thought that the surges of adrenaline due to the alcohol and partying lead to the development of the arrhythmia.

The most common arrhythmia associated with holiday heart is atrial fibrillation. The symptoms of palpitations and irregular heartbeat are most common. A person may feel weak, dizzy, short of breath, nauseated and they may even pass out. Prompt medical attention is necessary to assess the condition and be sure that no other severe medical problem is present.

ALCOHOL/DRUGS

WHAT IS THE TREATMENT? Most importantly, with issues concerning the heart, prompt medical attention is essential. It may be necessary to call 911 and arrive at the hospital by ambulance. As with most cases involving the heart, a comprehensive workup involving blood work, EKGs and x-rays will be ordered. As always, a complete history will be taken by your health care provider to assess other problems.

Once it is determined that a patient is suffering from holiday heart and they are stable, no treatment may be provided. Depending on the condition of the patient, some medications used to treat atrial fibrillation may be given. In the worst situation when a patient is unstable, cardioversion– a low dose electrical shock– will be used to get the patient back into a normal heart rhythm.

With holiday heart, the arrhythmia will usually resolve within 24 hours without treatment. Watchful waiting may be necessary while under medical care. With holiday heart, the condition will resolve on its own. There are no known residual effects.

Even though there are no long-lasting complications, the patient must assess their lifestyle and alcohol intake. This may be a warning sign of a potential problem. It is important to take this condition seriously.

So drink sensibly and monitor your alcohol intake. Cessation from drinking will help prevent the recurrence of holiday heart. Usually, that is the only necessary remedy.

Practice a healthy lifestyle during the holidays and throughout the year. If you feel that you have developed a holiday heart, you must seek medical attention to rule out any other underlying medical or cardiac problems. Early intervention will lead to a better outcome and a much happier holiday season!

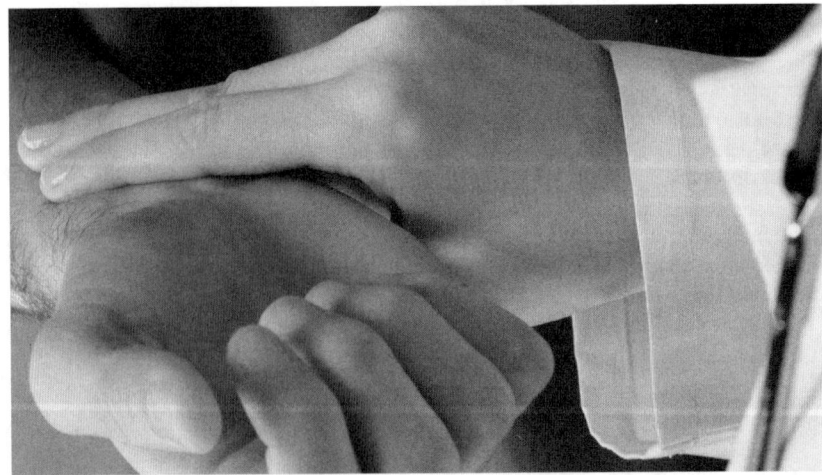

medication reconciliation

To address quality in health care, National Patient Safety Goals have been set forth by the accrediting body of hospitals and clinics. One of these goals has been medication reconciliation.

Over the past couple of years, statistics have shown that at least 350 medication errors have occurred in health care institutions and resulted in a major disability or death of the patient. All of these errors could have been prevented and the responsibility has been on the provider and the patient. Thus, most hospitals and clinics throughout the country are now involved in this initiative, and as a patient, you must help!

WHAT IS MEDICATION RECONCILIATION? This is a process that involves physicians, nurses, pharmacists and patients wherein the current medications are placed in an accurate list showing dosage and administration times. The list is reconciled with each step of the visit process in the hospital or at your doctor's office.

For example, a correct listing of medications is started in the emergency department upon arrival. That list is reconciled at the time of the discharge from the emergency department and would include any new medication prescribed. If the patient is discharged from the emergency department to the hospital, the medications are reconciled in the hospital and throughout the stay. When discharged after hospitalization, the patient will go home with a new, accurate list.

On an outpatient basis, the list should be brought to your physician office visit, as the medications will again be reconciled. This process keeps an accurate account of all medications that are being taken.

WHAT IS RECONCILED? The process involves the correct name and spelling of the medication. Several medications may sound alike and the correct one needs to be listed. Next, the proper dosage including number and unit of dosage must be checked. In addition, if new medications are added, interactions are checked and the prescriber is alerted to a potential harmful interaction.

ALCOHOL/DRUGS

Prescribed medications, vitamins, herbal medications and over-the-counter medications are all evaluated and checked. It should be noted that there are many harmful interactions between some herbal and over-the-counter medications and their prescriptive counter parts.

WHAT SHOULD I DO? As a patient, you have the responsibility to help ensure your own safety. You must provide your health care provider with the most accurate information as possible. It is important to know what medications and dosages you are taking.

It is impossible for your health care provider to know what you are taking when you state that it is "the little blue pill for my heart." Take a look in the Physicians Desk Reference and you will see several pills in different categories that fit the description. Also, it is not good practice to rely on your doctor to remember what you are taking.

Thus, when you go to the clinic or hospital for an appointment, take all of your prescribed and over-the-counter medications with you. This will allow the staff to evaluate what you are taking and provide an accurate list upon discharge.

Carry the accurate list with you at all times. Be sure this is the most current list and it is legible. If you are a nonmedical professional and are transcribing this list to your own document, be sure that you have included the proper dosage and the correct unit.

If you do not know your medications, your medical care may be delayed because the physician's office must call the pharmacy. If the medical visit occurs after pharmacy business hours, the data is not accessible. It is a good idea to purchase your medications from one source, as this contributes to consistency. It is also helpful for family members to assist in this process and know where medications are kept, along with a current list. This is very helpful when an emergency occurs.

Safety in health care is a huge initiative. National organizations are now monitoring this process and mandates are in place. Please help in this process to ensure that you receive the best health care possible. This simple process will make a difference in the delivery of quality health care. As providers, we continue to improve health care, but as a patient, you are also responsible for ensuring that you receive appropriate and safe care.

narcotics addiction

Americans were surprised to hear that one of America's most conservative and outspoken radio and TV personalities, Rush Limbaugh, had a narcotics addiction. Over the years, we have heard of numerous high-profile personalities with drug dependence problems. We have watched some of these individuals successfully complete treatment programs and remain clean, as others have had relapses and treatment failures.

This disease is not limited to high profile TV personalities and athletes, but can affect all people from a variety of socioeconomic levels. You may be surprised to learn that there are numerous individuals in your community with a dependence problem.

WHAT IS A NARCOTICS ADDICTION? Narcotics are strong prescription pain relievers that are considered controlled substances by the Drug Enforcement Administration (DEA). In addition to a medical license, health care providers must obtain an additional license to prescribe these medications.

Narcotics are used to control pain and they alter a patient's response to sensation. In addition, they may alter moods, change awareness or cause unconsciousness. If used improperly or mixed with other substances, death may occur.

Examples of narcotics include morphine, dilaudid, hydrocodone (Vicodin), heroin, methadone or meperidine (Demerol). Most of these medications are used effectively to manage pain, but repeated use leads to tolerance and eventual dependence.

HOW DOES THIS OCCUR? Over 70 million Americans suffer from some form of chronic pain. The causes of pain may come from a variety of sources and 1 in 5 people take a pain medicine on a daily basis. There are a variety of ways to treat chronic pain, including the use of medication or psychotherapy.

One of the mainstays to chronic pain management is the use of narcotics. Narcotics can be a very effective way to manage chronic pain, but a qualified health care provider must monitor their use.

WHO IS AT RISK FOR DRUG DEPENDENCE? A wide variety of factors may contribute to a drug dependence problem. Risk factors for the development of narcotics addiction include low self-esteem, environment, heredity, personality, types of drugs that have been used, and the ease of access to narcotics.

At present, Oxycontin, an oral form of morphine, is one of the most commonly abused narcotics. It is also one of the most common drugs that drug dealers attempt to obtain from health care providers through illicit and untruthful means. This is frustrating for clinicians, as it may be difficult to sort out real pain issues with some patients.

WHAT ARE SIGNS AND SYMPTOMS? The signs and symptoms of drug dependence are varied and may be nonspecific. If a clinician suspects excessive narcotics use by a patient, the issue must be addressed. Other clues may be some physical findings of constipation, alterations in vital signs, altered mental status or even signs of withdrawal.

Effects of narcotics may last a few days and signs of withdrawal may occur after several days of being drug-free. It is essential to admit that a problem exists and prepare for rehabilitation.

HOW IS DRUG DEPENDENCE TREATED? Once the problem has been identified, the patient must admit that the problem exists and consent to treatment. If the drug-dependent patient does not fully consent to treatment, the program is doomed to failure.

Treatment programs involve both medical and psychological facets. Patients may require hospital admission for detoxification, which may require additional use of medications to control withdrawal symptoms. Counseling needs to be initiated in the hospital and then carried out in the outpatient setting.

Programs such as Narcotics Anonymous are very helpful and emphasize a complete change in lifestyle. It is essential that a drug-free environment be maintained around the home.

WHAT ELSE SHOULD I DO? In the event that you suffer from a chronic pain condition, you must obtain adequate and comprehensive treatment. It is essential to have your primary care physician direct all of your care. Several different types of medications and therapies are available for treating chronic pain.

It is essential to stay away from illegal drugs. Do not use another person's medication. Be honest with your health care provider. Lastly, if you feel that you suffer from a narcotic addiction problem, admit it and seek treatment!

toxicology

After 9/11, as I sat in the toxicology review session of an emergency medicine board review course in Las Vegas, the Transportation Safety Association announced the ban of carry-on liquids on commercial aircraft. I received reports of three-to four-hour lines in order to get through security at McCarran International Airport. Fortunately, by early afternoon, I was able to traverse the maze of people and get to my gate in 90 minutes, which was about double the usual time for that airport.

It seems that terrorism is on everyone's mind and one form of terrorism may involve the use of poisonous substances. Since I last took my emergency medicine boards ten years ago, a few things have changed. With that said, I thought that I would discuss some of the most current concepts in dealing with poisoning.

WHAT IS TOXICOLOGY? This is the study of the adverse effects that chemicals have on living organisms. The evaluation of symptoms, mechanisms of injury, detection and treatment is the focus. A toxicologist is usually a physician that has completed fellowship training after residency. Many toxicologists are also emergency physicians. A great deal of my practice is spent on evaluating and treating the effects of accidental and intentional poisonings.

As I prepare to re-certify in emergency medicine, I am spending a great deal of time studying the most current treatments for a variety of poisonings caused by household chemicals and medicines. Many of the cases that are seen in the emergency department are intentional, but there are considerable accidental cases.

WHAT ARE THE PRINCIPLES OF TOXICOLOGY? Over the years, as health care providers, we have attempted to reduce exposure to poisons and increase safety. Treatment has been directed at reducing the absorption of poisons and increasing elimination from the body. Follow-up care has included supportive care either in the outpatient or hospital setting. Lastly, certain poisons and medications have specific treatment protocols that may include antidotes.

A large percentage of accidental poisonings involve children; one-half of these cases are secondary to medications. Overall, poisons with the highest mortality in children include cocaine, antidepressants, anticonvulsants and iron. The incidence of iron poisoning was a problem in the 1990s, but changes in packaging and volume have diminished this incidence.

HOW HAS INITIAL TREATMENT CHANGED? In the past, ipecac, a medicine that makes one vomit, was considered a standard household first aid treatment. It is not available at the drug store for over the counter purchase any longer. If you have some in your medicine cabinet, get rid of it. The medical literature has shown that it's dangerous to use and does not improve outcomes but actually interferes with actual treatment.

I am sure that many of you remember or have heard of someone having their stomach pumped in the emergency department. This used to be standard practice when I started working in the emergency department over 15 years ago. Stomach pumping, called gastric decontamination, has now been shown to have no benefit. Several medical studies have shown that this aggressive medical procedure can be quite dangerous and does not improve the end result.

Now, the mainstay of treatment is activated charcoal, which absorbs the poison or medicine. The charcoal acts as a sponge and binds with the offending product. Some charcoal preparations have additives that help with elimination through bowel cleansing. This should be given strictly under the direction of a health care provider.

WHAT SHOULD BE DONE WHEN A POISONING OCCURS?
Keep the patient safe, do not give ipecac, and call your local Poison Control Center. I recommend having the toll free number for your regional Poison Control Center available and displayed in a prominent spot, such as your refrigerator. The poison control specialists will give initial treatment advice, but be prepared to be directed to seek medical attention at your local emergency department. Poison Control will usually call the hospital to notify of the impending arrival.

Be sure to gather as much information as possible to assist the emergency department staff in identifying the poison or medication. Be sure to utilize your 911 EMS system in receiving help and getting to the hospital. This is important in life-threatening conditions.

As we are faced with a heightened terrorism alert, we need to be prepared to deal with toxicological emergencies. We must not overlook the common situations that occur in the home.

hypothyroid

A friend has asked that I discuss hypothyroidism, as a family member was recently diagnosed with this condition. This fairly common problem affects more women than men and is sometimes referred to as a goiter problem.

WHAT IS HYPOTHYROIDISM? This is a condition when the thyroid gland does not produce enough thyroid hormone. The thyroid gland is a butterfly-shaped organ that is located in the lower neck around the Adam's apple or larynx. It is small and weighs about an ounce.

The hormones produced by the thyroid are the T3 and T4 hormones. They are responsible for the regulation of metabolism, which includes how fast your heart beats, how fast you breathe or how quickly you burn off calories. Problems can arise from the gland itself, or from other associated organs in the brain such as the hypothalamus or the pituitary.

Usually, women over the age of 40 are more affected than men. It is interesting to note that about 17 percent of all women over the age of 60 will be affected by an under-active thyroid. The onset of the symptoms is fairly slow, but left untreated, an individual is at risk for numerous health problems.

WHAT ARE THE SYMPTOMS? There are several very nonspecific symptoms that are associated with hypothyroidism. These may include weakness, fatigue, cold intolerance, constipation, weight gain, depression, muscle pain and thinning nails along with brittleness of the hair. These can be early symptoms and if there are no other causes, this diagnosis should be entertained.

Later signs and symptoms include a slowed speech, dry skin, puffy face and hands, thinning of the eyebrows, and hoarseness. Further deterioration will lead to a severe condition called myxedema. The condition is very critical and death may occur.

WHAT ARE THE CAUSES? There are several causes for hypothyroidism and one of the most common is when the body actually attacks the thyroid gland through an autoimmune process. The body's immune system will irritate the thyroid gland and it becomes inflamed. This condition is called Hashimoto's

AUTOIMMUNE

thyroiditis. It is not clear why the body's immune system attacks itself. Ultimately, the thyroid gland is unable to produce the thyroid hormones due to the injury from the process.

Other causes of hypothyroidism include treatment with radioactive iodine or radiation. With an overactive thyroid, these medications are used to stop production of the thyroid hormones, thereby damaging the gland. With this treatment, the gland is unable to produce thyroid hormones. So the treatment of one condition leads to another condition.

Other causes include surgery to the thyroid to remove a growth that may lead to the gland's inability to produce the hormones, and medications that may damage the gland. One fairly common medicine that causes problems with the thyroid is Lithium, which is used to treat a bipolar psychiatric disorder.

Being over the age of 40 puts one at greater risk for hypothyroidism. There is also a hereditary component. Diabetes increases the risk for development of the disease.

HOW IS IT DIAGNOSED? In the event that you are experiencing the above symptoms, medical attention should be sought. A physical examination will lead the clinician to further investigate the situation. The simplest way to diagnose the problem is through a blood test to evaluate the levels of T3 and T4 hormones. Also, a check of the thyroid-stimulating hormone (TSH) is essential. This is all very important information for your health care provider.

WHAT IS THE TREATMENT? Once the condition is identified, a synthetic hormone will be prescribed. This is a levothyroxine called Synthroid. Life-long therapy will be necessary. The hormone levels will need to be monitored several times a year through a blood test.

A patient will start to feel better shortly after the treatment is initiated. The health care provider will need to monitor the dosages and make adjustments accordingly. Overall, a patient can expect a return to a normal, healthy lifestyle.

Hypothyroidism cannot be prevented. Awareness of the signs and symptoms are important. The severe untreated consequences can be avoided if medical attention is sought in a very timely fashion.

multiple sclerosis

In Wisconsin, over 10,000 patients receive services for multiple sclerosis (MS). The National Multiple Sclerosis Society provides research, education and assistance to these patients. MS usually affects patients in the prime of their life between the ages of 20 to 50. The effects can range from minor to debilitating.

WHAT IS MULTIPLE SCLEROSIS? MS is a disease of the central nervous system, that includes the brain and the spinal column. The myelin, which is the insulation over the nerve, deteriorates in certain areas. The breakdown of the insulation shows changes that are referred to as plaques. Also, the axon, which is the fiber that carries nerve impulses away from the nerve cell, will deteriorate and interfere with a normal nerve impulse.

There are two major types of MS. The first is more common whereby the symptoms experienced by the patient will wax and wane over a few days to weeks. Then, the symptoms will quiet down for a while. A more serious form of MS is called primary progressive disease whereby the symptoms will present and continue to worsen without a period of remission. This form only affects about 10 percent of the patients with MS.

WHAT ARE THE SYMPTOMS? The symptoms of MS can be very vague and nonspecific. Many patients seek medical attention several times before the diagnosis is made. Initially, a person may experience exhaustion, generalized weakness and increased clumsiness. There may be some blurred vision and generalized numbness and tingling. Then, these symptoms may go away for a while.

The hallmark of MS that clues your health care provider into an evaluation for MS is double vision. Once again, it should be noted that this might be accompanied by limb weakness, muscle stiffness, memory loss and depression. It is important to remember that these are very generalized symptoms that can be seen with all sorts of ailments.

AUTOIMMUNE

WHO IS AFFECTED? A majority of patients affected are between the ages of 20 to 40 years. MS is rarely diagnosed in children or people over the age of 60 years. Women are affected twice as many times as males. Family history of MS does increase the chances for development, but not by much. The disease is present worldwide and there are about a quarter million people living with MS in the United States.

WHAT IS THE CAUSE? There is no known cause of MS. It has been thought that this may be an autoimmune process. This means that the body may view the myelin as a foreign substance and destroy it. There is ongoing research to better identify the cause, but at the present time, the cause is still somewhat of a mystery. It is thought that stress and trauma may trigger the disease process of symptoms and remission.

HOW IS IT DIAGNOSED? Since the symptoms are vague, it may take your health provider a little time to make the diagnosis. MS is somewhat a diagnosis of exclusion because of the vague symptoms. The diagnostic test of choice is magnetic resonance imaging (MRI). An MRI of the brain will show some classic changes that are consistent with MS, showing the damaged myelin. It is important to remember that an MRI cannot be ordered on every person that presents with fatigue and weakness, so it may take a little time to rule out the disease process. Usually blood work will not help in making the diagnosis.

WHAT IS THE TREATMENT? Unfortunately, there is no cure for MS. There are a wide variety of medications that are being used to slow the progression of the process and increase the times of remission. Experimental treatments are being evaluated as well. Some of the most common treatments include steroids, Interferon, Copaxone, and intravenous immunoglobulins.

WHAT ELSE CAN BE DONE? Patients with MS need ongoing emotional support, in addition to the appropriate medical treatment. A team approach to the disease is essential and the team should consist of physicians, nurses, physical therapists, occupational therapists, social workers and counselors. This comprehensive plan can yield a fairly fulfilling life for the patient and the family.

rheumatoid arthritis

Since my dad was diagnosed with rheumatoid arthritis a couple of years ago, I find myself drawn to articles concerning RA.

In Australia, the health ministry finally approved the use of Remicade for sufferers of RA. This drug has been used in the United States over the past several years with great success. Aussies will now have the luxury of being treated with a highly-effective medication.

In the Netherlands, a new RA treatment study was released that was highly effective in rats. The regimen involves coating the anti-inflammatory steroid dexamethasone with a fat cell. The coated steroid is then effectively delivered to the sites of joint inflammation. The availability of this treatment for humans is probably several years away, if it is found safe and effective.

Let's take a closer look at RA, a disease that afflicts about 1 percent of all Americans usually diagnosed between the ages of 30 to 50.

WHAT IS RHEUMATOID ARTHRITIS? This is a chronic medical condition that destroys the joints and is a very specific type of arthritis. We are all familiar with osteoarthritis, known as "wear and tear" arthritis. This arthritis affects most individuals that have maintained an active life style, but is not the same as RA.

With RA, the sac surrounding the joint, called the synovium, becomes inflamed and eventually destroyed. As this protective joint sac is destroyed, so is the cartilage or protective tissue in the joint. As the joint becomes inflamed, it becomes narrowed. The bone in this area will be damaged and even destroyed. This leads to a disruption of joint function and obvious deformity. The soft tissue will thicken and harden, leading to an enlarged, deformed and painful joint. With severe disease, the joint may actually become dislocated.

WHAT IS THE CAUSE? The exact cause for the body attacking itself is not completely known. It is thought that there may be a large combination of factors that include abnormal immunity, genetics, environment and viral infections.

It is known that an autoimmune response occurs whereby the body begins an inflammatory response against itself. Genetic and hereditary factors are present, but do not play a strong role. It has been thought that some exposure to chemicals may place a person at risk. It should be noted that silicone breast implants, once thought to be a risk, do not lead to the development of RA. Lastly, some intestinal bacterial infections and viral infections may stimulate the autoimmune process, but this is not conclusive.

HOW IS THIS DIAGNOSED? To a certain degree, this is a clinical diagnosis. A patient may present with generalized aches and pains and the health care provider may be suspicious for RA. With more advanced cases, the presence of joint inflammation and swelling may be seen in the hands and feet. There may be significant joint abnormalities and the fingers and toes may have developed poor alignment. X-Rays will reveal some classic findings that will be followed up with lab testing. There are a variety of blood tests that will confirm the presence of the disease. With advanced disease, other body parts may become involved such as the spine, hips, skin, eyes, lungs, heart and gastrointestinal tract.

WHAT IS THE TREATMENT? Physical measures may involve protecting the joints and preventing further destruction. Goals of treatment involve preventing inflammation and further joint destruction. Preservation of movement is essential.

A wide variety of medications are used in the treatment of RA. Initially, non-steroidal anti-inflammatory medications are used, like ibuprofen. Corticosteroids such as prednisone and dexamethasone prevent acute flare-ups. The newer COX-II inhibitors like Celebrex are effective and may initially be prescribed.

More aggressive medications may be used such as the DMARDs (Disease Modifying Anti-Rheumatic Drugs), which include methotrexate. Lastly, the biggest breakthroughs in this treatment are medications called Tumor Necrosis Factor Modifiers. Two popular medications include Remicade and Enbrel, which are advertised on television to the general public.

WHAT ELSE SHOULD BE DONE? If you suspect that you suffer from RA, you should see your health care provider. A comprehensive evaluation of your history and a physical examination will be in order. Treatment should begin promptly, as the disease process must be stopped in order to help the patient continue to lead an active lifestyle.

hemolytic-uremic syndrome (HUS)

In Florida, over a dozen children were hospitalized with a near-fatal medical condition that was thought to be caused by visiting a petting zoo at a local state fair and a strawberry festival. This was the only common link for these children, who had a severe bacterium in their colon. This lead to trouble with their blood and kidneys. The diagnosis is Hemolytic-Uremic Syndrome (HUS). This is a fairly uncommon medical condition that affects children.

WHAT IS HUS? HUS is a condition that affects the blood cells, blood vessels and kidneys of children usually under the age of 10. The blood begins to clot and the platelets in the blood are also affected. There is damage within the blood vessels which eventually leads to damage of the small vessels of the kidneys, causing kidney failure. Children may become very sick and a small percentage may even die. Most children will recover, but they are at risk for developing permanent kidney damage.

WHAT CAUSES HUS? HUS is caused by exposure to a bacterium called E. Coli. There are many different strains of E. Coli and this offender is the OH157:H7 strain. This strain is found in the gut of cows, horses and sheep. It is important to remember that humans have E. Coli in their gut, but it is a different strain. Also, one of the most common bacteria that cause a bladder infection are E. Coli, but it is unrelated to the animal strain.

In Florida, the only common link between the affected children was a petting zoo at a county fair and a strawberry festival. Most likely, the children were interacting with the animals and became infected. It is a little more unlikely that they became infected from a common food source such as uncooked meat or infected milk. Usually, this is how children become infected. But the cases in Florida have alerted us to the potential dangers of exposure to animals in petting zoos.

BACTERIAL

WHAT ARE THE SYMPTOMS? Infected children will usually present with symptoms that are similar to the stomach flu. Children may develop abdominal pain, vomiting and diarrhea. The clue that something more serious is wrong is when the condition does not improve. Children may develop bloody diarrhea after about three days and this is cause for concern. Some children may appear somewhat ill and quite pale, even though the acute symptoms have resolved. The initial course may last from 1 to 15 days.

As the disease progresses and the blood begins to clot, the blood vessels may become damaged. This may lead to involvement of the kidney. There may be decreased urine output. Severe cases of kidney failure may lead to altered states of consciousness. In addition, parents may notice some unusual bruising on the skin of their sick child.

WHAT IS THE DIAGNOSIS AND TREATMENT? Children that have the above symptoms must be evaluated. Ill-appearing children mandate a workup by the health care provider. Granted, every case of stomach flu does not require medical attention, but if there are risk factors for a more serious disease or if the clinical course just does not seem right, the child must be evaluated.

The health care provider must assess the risks for the development of HUS, such as exposure to raw meat, petting zoos or other infectious illnesses. Physical examination may reveal some of the associated findings listed above. Laboratory assessment of the blood and kidneys is essential.

Most cases of HUS require appropriate evaluation, supportive therapy and sometimes hospitalization. More severe cases may require kidney dialysis or medications such as vincristine or cyclosporine. Additional types of blood therapies may be instituted as well.

WHAT IS THE OUTLOOK? About 85 to 90 percent of all children will recover without incident. A very small percentage is at risk for death. Early diagnosis is important, as well as good hygiene in order to prevent the development of HUS. More information can be found at www. kidney.org.

lyme disease

SARS, West Nile, Rotavirus– are we ever going to be free from concerns over catching a virus? Just when you ask the question, we're reminded of an old favorite that popped up in the early 90s: Lyme disease. To think when we first heard about this mysterious disease, there were so many unanswered questions. Now Lyme disease seems to be as common a summer health precaution as the flu is in winter. And just like the flu, we are able to protect ourselves. It is just a matter of familiarizing ourselves with what Lyme disease is and what precautions need to be taken to prevent it.

WHAT IS LYME DISEASE? Lyme disease is an infection transmitted by the bite of a deer tick — these ticks live in a warm, humid environment. The disease is actually named after Lyme, Connecticut, where it was first diagnosed in 1977. Initially, it presents as a rash, due to an inflammation of the vessels in the skin. If untreated, the infection can progress to infect the nervous system, which includes the brain. Also, if left untreated, the infection can affect the heart, causing an irregular heartbeat.

WHAT ARE THE SYMPTOMS? The symptoms of Lyme disease can be very vague and mimic other diseases. Most often, it involves a red, flat rash at the site of a recent tick bite. It may look like a red bull's eye surrounded by a target. Many times, the rash can be quite large and widespread. It may be in one spot, or there may be many blotches. Studies show that up to 90 percent of infected patients get this tell-tale rash, which can take up to a week or longer to appear after the tick bite. This part of the infection is considered to be in the early, localized stage.

If not diagnosed and treated early, other symptoms may develop, including fatigue, fever, headache, joint pain and general body aches. If left untreated, serious late-stage complications can include heart arrhythmias, confusion and severe, debilitating arthritis, which can lead to chronic arthritis.

AM I AT RISK? Risk for Lyme disease infection is dependent upon the geographic region where you may have been exposed. Ticks infected with Lyme disease are found primarily in three regions of the country — the Northeast, the Upper Midwest and the Upper Northwest. Over 80 percent of the diagnosed cases of Lyme disease come from these regions.

BACTERIAL

If you think that you've been bitten by a deer tick, have a rash and have spent time in any of these regions of the country, be sure to see your doctor for a blood test.

HOW IS IT TREATED? Based on the blood test results and a complete history of your recent activities, treatment may consist of prescribed medications. Antibiotics are the standard treatment. Recent studies have shown that patients who have a known deer tick bite from a high-risk area of the country may be effectively treated with one or two doses of antibiotics. Patients who are diagnosed with additional symptoms in the later stages of the disease will receive a longer course of antibiotics that may last two to three weeks.

Patients with the most severe symptoms may require hospitalization and IV antibiotics. Oftentimes, these patients are started on IV therapy in the hospital and then need to return as an outpatient on a daily basis for continued antibiotic treatment.

WHAT CAN I DO? If you live or vacation in a high-risk area, take appropriate precautions. Wear light-colored clothing and check yourself for ticks after spending time outside. Do a full body check on yourself and family members before going to bed every night. Also, consider using an insect repellent with DEET (diethylmetatoluamide) and avoid sitting directly on the ground. You can also help to "tick proof" your yard by keeping it well groomed and keeping wood piles neatly stacked.

Remember, the symptoms of Lyme disease can be very vague, but the appearance of a rash after being bitten by an insect can be a tell-tale sign, so be sure to see your doctor.

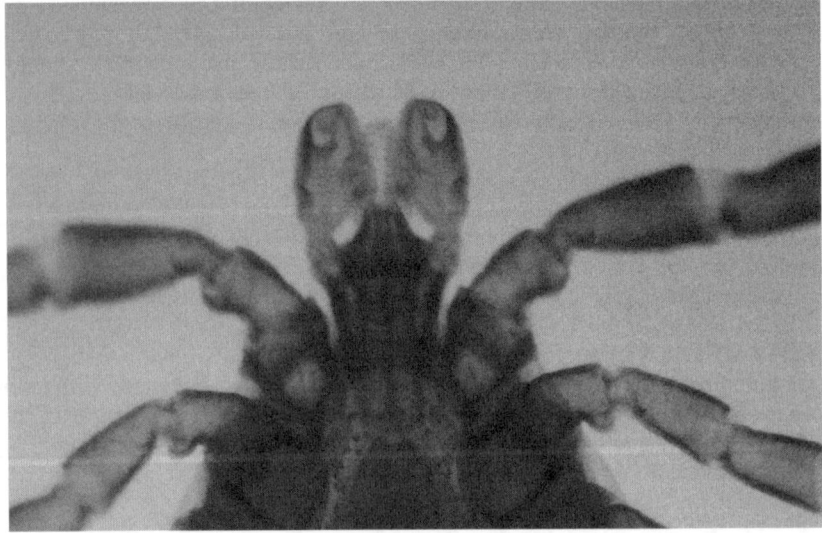

To Your Health with Dr. Wojo

meningitis

A deceptive, rapidly-progressing and sometimes fatal disease is jeopardizing the lives of children and college students throughout America. This silent stalker is often mistaken for the flu, but if left untreated meningitis can turn deadly. Sharing the same common bacteria (streptococcus pneumonia) found in ear infections, blood infections and pneumonia, meningitis is a serious disease process.

But according to a recent study by the Centers for Disease Control (CDC), childhood vaccinations for pneumococcal meningitis work. This CDC study also proves that the racial gap of meningitis, which is more prevalent among black children, has been significantly reduced due to immunization.

WHAT IS MENINGITIS? Meningitis is an infection of the cerebral spinal fluid (CSF) that surrounds the brain and the spinal cord. A virus most commonly causes the infection. These cases are milder in form with less serious consequences. Usually, no specific treatment is required.

The second most common source of infection is due to several bacterias, including Streptococcus pneumonia, Haemophilus influenzae and Neisseria meningitides. The result of this infection can lead to brain damage and learning disabilities if not treated with appropriate antibiotics in a timely fashion.

WHAT ARE THE SYMPTOMS? The most common symptoms in children and adults may include headaches, fever and a stiff neck. There may be an associated respiratory illness prior to the development of meningitis. As the disease progresses in severity, there may be confusion, loss of consciousness, nausea, vomiting and a very ill appearance. Lastly, a person with meningitis may become combative or experience seizures. It is important to look at the big clinical picture, as many of the symptoms can be present with numerous other medical conditions.

HOW IS THE DIAGNOSIS MADE? Your health care provider must be suspicious of meningitis on the basis of the clinical presentation and risk factors present. In addition, exposure to other people with some forms of meningitis increases the chance of developing meningitis. The presence of a respiratory illness, ear infection, sinusitis, or pneumonia are major risks for the spread of the infection to the CSF.

BACTERIAL

Once your health care provider is suspicious for meningitis, blood work and x-rays may be completed. A CT scan of the head may be ordered to check for the presence of an infectious process in the brain. Finally, a lumbar puncture or spinal tap will be completed to look for the evidence of an infectious process, either viral or bacterial, in the CSF.

A lumbar puncture is a very safe and fairly painless procedure that is done in the prone or seated position. The lower back is cleansed and anesthetized. A small needle is passed in between the vertebrae to obtain the fluid. The fluid is then sent to the laboratory for microscopic analysis and culture. The culture may take a couple of days to reveal the offending bacteria. Viral cultures are usually not ordered because by the time the results are in, the patient has fully recovered.

WHAT IS THE TREATMENT? Viral meningitis requires only supportive treatment and most patients will improve within a couple of days. Several of these cases are admitted to the hospital in order to be sure that the infection is viral in nature.

Bacterial meningitis is a very serious condition and prompt treatment with intravenous antibiotics is necessary. Some cases require the use of steroids as well. Hospitalization is mandatory and very close follow-up is required. Meningococcal meningitis, which is a specific bacterium, requires that all who come into contact with the patient be given a single dose of an oral antibiotic. This is the infection that has occurred in some university dorm settings and has lead to the unfortunate deaths detailed in national media headlines.

WHAT ELSE SHOULD I DO? It is important to have children immunized. This simple preventative measure can prevent the development of many forms of bacterial meningitis. Be sure that your children are up-to-date on their shots, as you can decrease the possibility of your children developing a potentially life-threatening infection that can also lead to a permanent disability.

For more information on meningitis and support services for victims of meningitis, visit the Meningitis Foundation of America website at www.musa.org.

methicillin-resistant
staphylococcus
aureus
(MRSA)

Major concern has been raised in the United Kingdom over the growing incidence of methicillin-resistant Staphylococcus Aureus infections, that are commonly referred to as MRSA (pronounced mer-sa). This is not only a concern across the Atlantic, but also here in our own communities. A day does not pass in the emergency department when I do not encounter a patient who has been infected with MRSA. This is a significant health care issue that must be appropriately dealt with.

WHAT IS MRSA? Staph Aureus is the most common bacteria found in skin infections such as pimples or boils. In the past, these bacteria were very sensitive to common first-line antibiotics such as penicillin or cephalosporin. But, due to over-use of these antibiotics, through mutation the bacteria have rendered these antibiotics inactive. Unfortunately, doctors and patients are to blame. Physicians have over-prescribed antibiotics for a variety of conditions and patients have come to expect an antibiotic prescription for any hint of an infection, whether viral or bacterial.

The seriousness of the MRSA infection extends beyond the simple pimple. Hospitalized patients are now infected with this "super infection" that is invading the lungs, surgical sites and the blood stream. This mandates the use of the strongest antibiotics available in order to get rid of the infection. Sometimes a patient becomes much too sick to survive.

HOW COMMON IS MRSA? In the United States, there are about 100,000 cases of patients that are specifically hospitalized for the treatment of MRSA infections in wounds, blood stream or pneumonia. About 25-30 percent of all Americans are colonized or carriers of a basic Staph infection, with 1 percent being carriers of MRSA.

In the United Kingdom, the numbers are higher. A new strain of MRSA was identified in Ireland and a two-day-old child was treated for MRSA. This has heightened the awareness of health care officials in the UK.

BACTERIAL

WHAT DOES MRSA LOOK LIKE? From a gross clinical appearance, there are not distinguishing factors. A pimple or boil infected with MRSA looks like any other infection. So do other wound infections and pneumonias. The diagnosis is made in the laboratory under the microscope and on culture.

Pus is grown on a media and then exposed to different antibiotics. MRSA will grow in the presence of a variety of common antibiotics and be killed by very strong antibiotics. This process may take a couple of days to accomplish, and thus the health of the patient may deteriorate during this identification process. Why not use strong antibiotics initially? Well, this would contribute to the problem! It is important to use the right antibiotic to treat the infection.

WHO IS AT RISK? MRSA is more common in patients who have been hospitalized or live in a nursing home. Increased exposure to health care facilities and antibiotics places the patient at risk. Also, patients with chronic medical problems and who are immunocompromised by AIDS or cancer treatments are at significant risk. This is a growing problem in our healthy communities and community-acquired MRSA is on the rise. In 2003, about 12 percent of MRSA infections were community acquired.

WHAT SHOULD I DO TO PREVENT THE SPREAD OF MRSA?
Universal precautions are very important in the hospital setting to help control the spread of the infection. This involves good hand washing and the use of gloves. But, at home, it is important to do the same. If you have a wound, keep it covered until it is healed. Do not touch other people's open wounds. Do not share razors and towels. These simple measures can help in stopping the spread of the problem.

Lastly, it is very important to not pressure your health care provider into prescribing antibiotics when they are not necessary. As a physician, I want to be sure that my patients are satisfied with the treatment I provide. I attempt to explain the dangers of the inappropriate use of antibiotics, but this may take a lot of convincing on my part. Trust your health care provider and help in preventing the spread of a potentially life-threatening problem.

pertussis

There has been an increase in the number of cases of pertussis in the United States over the past couple of years. Pertussis, known as whooping cough, is a lower respiratory illness that is named for the way it sounds. It is most common in children, but can be seen in all age categories. Even though it is fairly uncommon, health care providers must think of this disease when confronted with a patient showing respiratory symptoms.

WHAT IS PERTUSSIS? Pertussis is a bacterial respiratory illness that is caused by Bordatella pertussis. The characteristic cough associated with this illness is very high-pitched and quite severe. Pertussis is also associated with other cold-like symptoms.

Pertussis was first diagnosed in the 16th century, but bacteria were not isolated in the laboratory until 1906. Until the mid-1940s, there were over 200,000 cases annually in the United States. After the development of the vaccine, that number began to steadily decline and by the early 1970s, there were only about 1,000 cases reported annually. Unfortunately, that number has begun to climb and the latest reports reveal an average of 4,000 annual cases.

WHAT ARE THE SYMPTOMS? The clinical features of whooping cough are divided into three stages. The first stage, or catarrhal stage, is characterized by a sudden onset of a runny nose, sneezing, mild cough, low fever and symptoms of a common cold. This usually occurs within 7 to 10 days after exposure and this initial stage may last up to two weeks. At the end of this stage, the cough becomes more violent.

The second stage is when the diagnosis of pertussis is usually made. By this time, the cough is quite severe and the patient experiences sudden bursts of coughing with associated difficulties in breathing. Thick mucous may be present as well. In addition, the coughing may be so severe that the patient may turn blue and vomiting may be precipitated. After the bout of coughing, the patient will look almost completely normal.

The final state or convalescent stage, is when recovery begins and may last weeks or months. The coughing fits decrease in intensity whereby they soon disappear. It is important to note that the fever is not usually very high, nor common during the course of the illness.

HOW IS IT DIAGNOSED? The early diagnosis of whooping cough may be difficult, as the initial presentation is similar to the common cold or influenza. Once the second stage of the illness is entered and the patient experiences the severe bouts of high-pitched coughing, the clinician must think of this disease.

Diagnosis is made by laboratory testing of a swab that is taken from the nasal passage, but the bacteria can be difficult to isolate. Clinicians must be suspicious of the disease on the basis of history, exposure, clinical presentation and laboratory findings.

WHAT IS THE TREATMENT? This respiratory illness requires supportive treatment and antibiotics. Once the diagnosis is suspected, erythromycin or sulfa should be prescribed. The antibiotic must be taken for its full course, which is usually 14 days. The confirmation of the culture revealing pertussis may take several days or weeks, so treatment is usually based on clinical suspicion.

Since pertussis is highly contagious, all household members that are exposed to the infected patient must be treated with antibiotics for 14 days as well. Unfortunately, about 20 percent of all infected and symptomatic patients require hospitalization for respiratory support and intravenous antibiotics. The most common associated complication is pneumonia. Fortunately, death is rare and occurs in less than 1 percent of all cases.

WHAT SHOULD I DO? Prevention is the best medicine. Immunization for pertussis is accomplished in children in their first two years of life through the administration of the DPT (Diphtheria-Pertussis-Tetanus) vaccination. It is essential that all children be immunized and this vaccine is very safe. Reactions and side effects to this shot are now minimal, and the protection far outweighs the risks. The risks and complications of pertussis are too great for people not to be immunized.

septic shock

Pope John Paul II suffered from failing health– including Parkinson's disease, respiratory failure and tracheotomy– which concluded with septic shock.

There are numerous types of shock that may result from trauma, brain injury, heart attack and blood loss. Septic shock is fairly common, but this is something that we do not hear about too frequently.

WHAT IS SEPTIC SHOCK? Septic shock is a form of shock that is caused by the presence of bacteria in the blood. When a person experiences "blood poisoning," numerous changes occur in the body. The blood pressure drops and the body is essentially deprived of appropriate blood flow and oxygen. Vital organs, such as the brain, heart, liver and kidneys begin to malfunction. All of these changes lead to a decline, eventually leading to death.

WHAT IS THE CAUSE? Septic shock results from sepsis, which is an over-whelming bacterial infection. The infection may start because of pneumonia, a skin infection, or bladder infection. With the Pope, it was thought that he had developed a bladder infection that eventually traveled to the blood stream.

When bacteria are present and they produce an infection, they release numer-ous toxins or poisons that aggravate the body's immune system. When these toxins are released in the blood stream, a whole series of events will occur. This includes the blood vessels dilating and lowering the blood pressure. The blood vessels are actually affected and they become leaky, allowing fluids to pass outside of the circulatory system. This leads to a lower blood pressure and less blood flow to a variety of body organs. Various organs are damaged due to the lack of blood flow.

WHO IS AT RISK? Septic shock usually occurs in the very young and the elderly. Many of these patients have an underlying medical condition that places them at risk. Some of these conditions include diabetes, leukemia, lymphoma, cancer, and poor immune systems secondary to disease or medicine, as well as recent surgical procedures.

BACTERIAL

WHAT ARE THE SYMPTOMS? Septic shock is usually preceded by an underlying infection. A patient may start with symptoms of fatigue, fever, chills, weakness and nausea. This may progress to a very high fever with rapid pulse rate, rapid breathing, diminished urination and low blood pressure.

As the disease state progresses, there is total organ failure including brain, kidney and liver. Eventually, a person becomes unconscious and is unable to recover.

HOW IS IT DIAGNOSED? Clinicians must be suspicious of septic shock in patients that experience a rapid deterioration after an infection. Blood tests and cultures will be taken. x-rays may help in localizing an infection. Also, evaluation of a urine sample must be completed, as this is a frequent source of infection.

WHAT IS THE TREATMENT? Initially, early diagnosis and recognition of an infection is important. Bacteria cause most cases of septic shock, but it can be caused by a viral or fungal infection as well. The offending bug should be identified and if bacterial, antibiotics should be promptly given.

As septic shock progresses, fluids will be given to raise the blood pressure. If a person does not respond to intravenous therapy, medicines may be added to increase the blood pressure. Patients may deteriorate very quickly and they may need to be placed on a ventilator. Use of oxygen is an important treatment. Newer drugs used to deal with the bacteria toxins may also be administered.

WHAT IS THE PROGNOSIS? The chance of dying from septic shock is over 50 percent, depending on the type of bug that is causing the infection and how quickly it is identified. Therefore, it is essential to seek prompt medical attention from your health care provider or the emergency department. The sooner one is treated, the greater the chance of survival. Timely treatment of an infection is helpful, but the development of septic shock may not be easily preventable.

syphilis

The CDC has recently reported nearly a 10 percent increase in the number of reported syphilis cases in the United States. This rise, occurring in the last two years, has been specifically noted in males and is attributed to males having sexual relations with other males; females may become infected.

WHAT IS SYPHILIS? Syphilis is a sexually transmitted disease caused by bacteria, called Treponema pallidum, through sexual contact. It has been called "the great imitator" over the years because of its nonspecific symptoms, which can be indistinguishable from other disease processes.

HOW DOES IT OCCUR? The bacteria are transmitted from person-to-person by direct contact and may enter the body through the mouth, rectum, vagina or a break in the skin. The bacteria are released from an infected individual and directed to another person, thereby infecting that person.

It is important to understand that it is not through contact with toilet seats, doorknobs, dinnerware, swimming pools, hot tubs or the sharing of clothing that one may become infected. Women may pass the infection to unborn children through the birth process. This is very serious, as the child may develop serious mental and physical problems, potentially resulting in death.

WHAT ARE THE SYMPTOMS? Syphilis presents in three stages and the primary stage occurs after 10 days of infection, lasting up to three months. The initial complaint may involve the development of a painless soft, reddened sore called a chancre (pronounced "shanker"). There may be one sore or multiple sores, but the first sore is where the syphilis has entered the body. There may be some other symptoms such as fever, body aches, swollen lymph nodes and loss of appetite. If untreated, the chancre will disappear.

With the second stage of the untreated disease, the latent phase, many of the physical signs and symptoms disappear; yet the disease can still be transmitted. Some patients may develop a rash on the palms and feet, which can mimic several other diseases. In addition, a person may continue to have non-specific complaints of fever, body aches and muscle pains. This stage may last for several months to several years.

BACTERIAL

The final stage, which is called late or tertiary syphilis, is very serious and results in permanent complications. These complications may include brain damage, blindness, deterioration of the nerves and blood vessels, bone and joint damage, as well as death. This may take several years to occur after the first infection, which is usually undiagnosed.

HOW IS IT DIAGNOSED? In the first stage, a health care provider must be suspicious of the sore and perform a scraping to look for the bacteria under a microscope. There is also a blood test that can be performed. Unfortunately, the blood test is not very sensitive in the early stages of the disease. It is extremely important for the health care provider to obtain a comprehensive history with regard to the exposure, which may include the sexual activity with other, possibly infected patients. Close observation must occur if the health care provider is suspicious.

HOW IS IT TREATED? The early stages of syphilis may be so mild that treatment may not be sought. Syphilis is sensitive to penicillin and is effectively treated with oral doses or shots. The ability to transmit the disease stops within 24 hours of treatment, as the penicillin is very effective in stopping the progression of the infection. Treatment is necessary for several days.

Ongoing testing and reassessment is necessary in order to be sure that the disease has been cured. Early treatment is necessary in order to prevent later complications. Unfortunately, if syphilis is left untreated and organ damage occurs, there is no reversing these permanent effects with penicillin.

WHAT SHOULD I DO? Prevention is the key, as with so many illnesses. Safe sexual activity is important in order to prevent this infection and other sexually transmitted diseases. In the event that you are suspicious of a sore and have participated in high-risk sexual activity, your health care provider must see you. You may prevent life-long health complications.

tuberculosis (TB)

Recently, the State Department suspended the immigration of Hmong refugees from the camps in Thailand due to a high incidence of tuberculosis (TB) infections among the immigrants. Cases of TB in the refugees have been diagnosed in California, Minnesota, and Wisconsin. I am sure that many of our older citizens remember the sanatoriums of the 1940s and 1950s that kept patients quarantined while being treated for TB. Today, TB is a fairly uncommon disease, but still present in small numbers in the United States.

WHAT IS TUBERCULOSIS? TB is a chronic bacterial (germ) infection that is caused by the organism called Mycobacterium tuberculosis. This bacteria will infect the lungs initially. They will eventually spread to other body parts including the kidneys, bones, spine and skin. Many people may actually harbor the bacteria, but will not have an active disease process.

WHAT IS THE INCIDENCE? In the 17th and 18th centuries, TB was very common in Europe and responsible for the "White Plague." During this time period, nearly 100 percent of the Europeans were infected and 25 percent died from TB. In the 1940s, the discovery of medicine lead to the treatment of this infectious process and by the early 1980s, TB was nearly unheard of in the United States.

Unfortunately, with the spread of AIDS and drug abuse, many people's immune systems were unable to fight off this infection, thereby increasing incidence rates from 1985 to 1992. Researchers and health care providers were aware of this, leading to appropriate diagnosis and treatment.

Worldwide, the incidence of TB is nearly 2 billion cases each year. About 2 to 3 million people die from this preventable disease. In the United States, there are only about 15,000 cases each year with a small percentage dying. The countries with the highest number of cases include Asia, Africa, and eastern Europe.

WHAT ARE THE SYMPTOMS? About 10 percent of the people who are infected with TB will develop an active disease process. The symptoms of TB include a severe cough lasting over two weeks, coughing up blood and pain in the chest. In addition, as the disease progresses, weight loss and fatigue may occur. Other symptoms include fever, chills and night sweats.

BACTERIAL

As you can see, the symptoms are very nonspecific and may mimic many other respiratory illnesses. Your health care provider must assess your risks, clinical course and presentation. The chances of getting TB are quite low, but your clinician must be suspect in unusual circumstances.

HOW IS THE DIAGNOSIS MADE? A clinical history assessing risks and symptoms is important. Routine testing is completed among a wide variety of professionals such as health care workers and educators. People living in close contact, such as nursing homes, must be screened. TB is spread from person to person by respiratory droplets, so this type of an environment can be a risk for an infected individual and other residents.

The screening process involves a TB skin test that is usually completed at the doctor's office. A small amount of the bacteria is injected under the skin and then the skin is re-evaluated after 72 hours. If there is a red welt at the injection site, the test is positive. A positive skin test does not always mean that a person has an active infection. The person may have been exposed and fought off the disease.

Follow-up testing may include a chest x-ray. In patients with a cough, the sputum or phlegm is cultured in the laboratory. It may take a month for this culture to grow out TB, as it grows very slowly. It is important to remember that infected patients with active TB are usually sick and have some respiratory symptoms.

WHAT IS THE TREATMENT? Prevention of the spread of the disease is essential. If you have an active case, you will need to stay home. Over the years, the TB bacteria has mutated (changed) and become quite strong. Resistance to some of the antibiotics used have occurred.

Today, most infected patients may have to take up to three antibiotics for up to six months to cure the infection. The most common antibiotics prescribed for TB include isoniazid (INH), rifampin, pyrazinamide, ethambutol, and streptomycin. Your provider will need to determine which medicines are best based on the resistance patterns in your community.

typhoid fever

It was interesting to watch news reports from France stating that Osama Bin Laden was dead of typhoid fever. Thinking about this disease took me back to my days in medical school studying for an infectious disease exam.

On my recent board recertification exams, I was not asked about typhoid fever, but my interest was piqued. I have never seen or treated a case and current statistics show that it is pretty rare in the United States. But, in the developing world, about 12.5 million cases are diagnosed each year. In the United States, there are about 400 cases annually, primarily from travelers that have returned from endemic areas.

WHAT IS TYPHOID FEVER? This is a life-threatening illness that is caused by the bacteria called Salmonella Typhi. The illness starts out as a high fever and "stomach flu," which progresses to a full systemic illness if left untreated.

With typhoid fever, a patient will become infected from food or beverages that have been handled by an infected person. Another risk of infection comes from drinking contaminated water or water that is used to wash foods. When the bacteria are ingested, they begin to multiply and eventually go into the blood stream.

The industrialized nations of the United States, Canada, Western Europe, Japan and Australia are low-risk countries. The high-risk countries are Asia, Africa and Latin America. Thus, travelers must be cautious when planning a trip to these areas.

WHAT ARE THE SYMPTOMS? Once a person is infected, they will develop a fever that may last for a week, before other symptoms start. It may take a week or more for symptoms to present once infected. Fevers are usually quite high, ranging in the 103-104° F range.

BACTERIAL

The next week of the illness consists of abdominal pain and the development of a rash. The rash is a faint salmon color that involves the trunk and abdomen. The appearance is referred to as macular, which looks like flat colored areas.

The third week of the illness leads to an enlarged spleen and liver, internal bleeding and infection. Patients will usually be confused and have an altered mental status. This stage can lead to death from the infection and organ failure.

WHAT IS THE TREATMENT? Once the diagnosis is made on the basis of clinical history, risk of exposure and symptoms, a stool culture will confirm the diagnosis. The treatment of choice will involve an antibiotic such as sulfa, penicillin or a fluoroquinolone. If treated in a timely fashion, a person will usually feel better in a couple of days. Typhoid is survivable without treatment, but only in individuals who are very healthy and do not have underlying medical problems. Full recovery without treatment may take several weeks to months.

WHAT ELSE SHOULD BE DONE? Prevention is the best practice when you are traveling. The CDC has the following recommendation, "Boil it, cook it, peel it, or forget it!" Thus, boil your water in an endemic area or drink bottled water. Be sure that your food is adequately cooked and served steaming hot. Only eat vegetables and fruits that you can peel yourself. This is all simple advice. Otherwise, forget it!

When you are traveling to a high-risk country, be sure to get the typhoid vaccine. It is highly effective in preventing Typhoid Fever, but it must be received at least a week in advance of the trip. Also, the vaccination does lose its effectiveness after time, so a booster will be necessary for return visits.

As is the case with so many medical conditions, you should seek attention if you are concerned. Also, be sure to seek medical advice from your health care provider when traveling to an endemic area. The Internet is a good source of reputable sites such as www.cdc.gov. You will find a wide variety of recommendations for travel and vaccinations.

Aspirin

"An aspirin a day will keep the doctor away." We have all heard that at least a thousand times. "Take two aspirin and call me in the morning." Even though these have been jokes for several decades, there is some truth and benefit to these simple treatments. A recent study from Germany has once again confirmed the fact that aspirin after a myocardial infarction or heart attack will reduce the chance of death by at least 50 percent in the first year. Aspirin is one of the most cost-effective treatments in medicine today. Aspirin is a fairly safe medication, but its use should be recommended and monitored by a health care provider. In general, the risks with the use of aspirin are less than the life-long benefits.

WHAT IS ASPIRIN'S MECHANISM OF ACTION? Aspirin works on the blood by affecting the actions of the platelets. Platelets are cells in the blood that help in the clotting process. Aspirin affects the ability of the platelets to stick together and form a clot. Therefore, someone taking aspirin will bleed a little longer.

The use of aspirin has implications in heart disease where blood vessels are narrowed. The narrowing of the blood vessel is called a plaque. With a narrowed vessel, blood can clot and block the vessel. The chances of blood clotting are diminished when one takes aspirin. This plays a role in preventing a heart attack or the recurrence of a heart attack. Therefore, life span is increased due to this simple, inexpensive medication.

IS THERE A RISK IN TAKING ASPIRIN? As with all medications, there can be side effects. Aspirin is known to place a patient at risk for increased bleeding–from simple cuts to internal bleeding. Patients taking aspirin are at greatest risk for developing bleeding in the stomach and intestinal tract. This can be a very serious and life-threatening problem.

If you suffer from high blood pressure, stomach ulcers, a bleeding disorder, had a stroke, have liver or kidney problems, asthma, or previous allergy, then aspirin should not be taken without medical supervision. If you have any of these health problems then you must consult your primary health care provider for advice on the use of aspirin.

BLOOD

Aspirin may also interact with other medications. It is really important to consult your medical provider or pharmacist to be sure that no problem exists with the use of aspirin. Additionally, the use of alcohol and aspirin raises the risk of bleeding. These are all very important considerations.

WHAT CONDITIONS DOES ASPIRIN HELP? Medical studies have shown time and time again that the use of aspirin can prevent the development of a heart attack in high-risk patients. It will also reduce the severity of heart damage during a heart attack and it also helps in reducing recurrence after a heart attack. Aspirin may also help in reducing angina, which is chest pain associated with heart disease.

When a person with heart disease undergoes cardiac catheterization, where the vessels on the heart are injected with dye and x-rayed, aspirin can prevent the development of clots after the procedure. This is especially important if a narrowed vessel is opened with a balloon.

In addition to heart problems, aspirin is very effective in treating brain problems such as mini-strokes know as transient ischemic attacks (TIA), or full blown strokes. In patients that have suffered a stroke, outcome and follow-up is improved with the use of aspirin.

WHEN SHOULD I TAKE ASPIRIN? Even though aspirin is a very inexpensive drug and readily available, it is important to discuss long-term usage with your health care provider. Taking it is not without risk. You will need to discuss how much to take and how frequently. The risks and benefits must be assessed. Overall, aspirin is one of the best values in medicine!

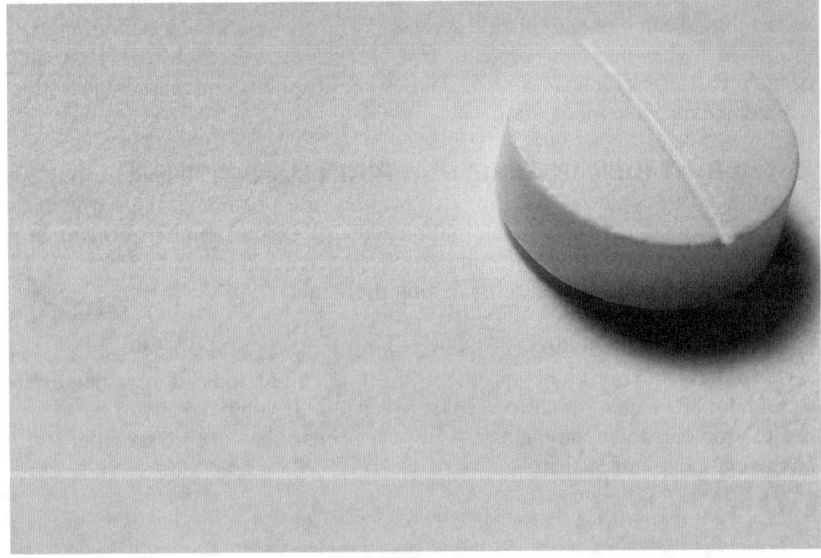

coumadin

Wisconsin has been on the leading front for many medical phenomena and now we can add one of the most talked about medicines to that list. The University of Wisconsin-Madison discovered Coumadin (Warfarin), the leading anticoagulant, in the country.

More and more people are finding themselves either driving to the local pharmacy, or taking that extended trip to Canada for reduced rates, to obtain Coumadin. It is one of the medicines currently on the market with the fewest restrictions, including the fact that you can take it on an empty or full stomach.

WHAT IS COUMADIN? Coumadin is a medicine that is referred to as a "blood thinner." In actuality, Coumadin does not thin the blood. It interrupts the body's natural processes during blood clotting, thereby increasing the time it takes for the blood to clot. In addition, it makes the body more susceptible to undesired bleeding.

Ultimately, Coumadin does not allow blood clots to form in blood vessels, and in the presence of a blood clot, it does not allow the clot to become bigger. Also, Coumadin does not allow blood clots to form in the chambers of a heart with heart beat irregularities called arrhythmias.

WHY IS IT PRESCRIBED? Coumadin is prescribed for a variety of medical conditions. The goal is to prevent blood clotting.

The most common use of Coumadin is to prevent the development of a blood clot in one of the heart chambers during a cardiac arrhythmia (irregular heart beat). The most common cardiac arrhythmia requiring the use of Coumadin is atrial fibrillation. Studies have shown that patients with atrial fibrillation can prevent 85 percent of strokes if they take Coumadin.

Another condition that warrants the use of Coumadin includes a pulmonary embolism (lung blood clot). These patients may be on Coumadin for six months after the diagnosis is made. Its use will prevent the development of further clots and the spread of old clots. Pulmonary emboli are very serious and can be fatal without the use of Coumadin, as blood clots in the lungs prevent oxygenation of the blood.

BLOOD

Patients that are at risk for stroke may be prescribed Coumadin. Also, patients with blood clots in the legs called deep venous thrombosis (DVT), will have to take Coumadin for at least a three-month period in order to prevent further clot development. These blood clots, when left untreated, can travel to the lungs. Finally, all patients with artificial mechanical heart valves must take Coumadin for the rest of their lives in order to prevent blood clots from forming on the valves.

HOW IS IT MONITORED? A patient taking Coumadin will generally have to have their blood checked monthly. Many clinics have developed a separate service managed by nurses to evaluate the amount of Coumadin that is taken based on lab studies. The test that is followed is the Prothrombin Time (PT) and the International Normalized Ratio (INR).

The PT measures the time it takes for the blood to clot and the INR is a standard that is used to account for differences between labs. This allows patients to have their blood tested at different labs and the physician is able to monitor the Coumadin with consistency.

In the event that Coumadin levels become too high, the medicine may be held back or Vitamin K may be administered. Patients must avoid foods high in Vitamin K, such as leafy green vegetables, which will interfere with the function of the Coumadin.

WHAT ARE THE SIDE EFFECTS? Excessive bleeding is the most common side effect of an elevated level of Coumadin. Patients are at risk for bruising as well. Other serious side effects may include the development of gastrointestinal bleeding from an ulcer or stomach irritation. Also, elevated Coumadin levels may contribute to blood in the urine. Any of these side effects can be life threatening and must be evaluated by your health care provider.

In conclusion, Coumadin is a life-saving drug. In general, it is very safe, but requires very close medical supervision. Patients need to be careful not to injure themselves by falling from a considerable height. It is not advisable to use alcohol when taking this medication. You and your health care provider must evaluate the risks, benefits and alternatives to its usage. Most importantly, if your doctor has prescribed Coumadin, do not stop taking it unless this action is approved!

deep venous thrombosis (DVT)

It is important to realize that a long car ride may put you at risk for a blood clot in your leg. A long plane ride may do the same. A blood clot in the leg is a very serious condition that can lead to a blood clot in the lungs, which can be fatal. A clot in the leg is called a Deep Venous Thrombosis (DVT).

WHAT IS A DVT? A DVT is a blood clot in the deep venous system of the legs. Most DVTs occur in the legs, but can occur in the arms as well. Veins are the blood vessels that return the blood back to the heart. These clots are dangerous because they can break off and travel to other parts of the body such as the lungs. When the clot is in the lungs, it is called a pulmonary embolism and can be a fatal condition.

HOW DOES IT OCCUR? During a prolonged period of immobility or activity, the blood in the legs will move more slowly through the veins and with this slower flow, the blood may begin to clot. Once the process of clotting is started, it begins to build up quite quickly, forming a large blood clot.

WHAT ARE THE RISK FACTORS FOR DVT? A prolonged period of inactivity can contribute to a blood clot in the lower extremity. This may include a long car ride or long plane ride. In general, it has been shown that eight hours of inactivity in cramped quarters such as a small car or in an airplane seat will increase the risk of a DVT.

Other conditions that can contribute to the development of a DVT include immobilization for a hip or pelvis fracture, cancer, heart disease, high blood pressure, obesity and blood disease. In addition, smoking is a major risk factor for the development of a clot.

WHAT ARE THE SYMPTOMS? Most commonly, a swollen painful leg is suggestive of a blood clot in the leg. Others signs that are worrisome include a warm leg with redness, cramps, or discoloration. It is interesting to note that half of all patients may not have any symptoms. It is important to assess the risk factors in association with the symptoms.

HOW IS A DVT DIAGNOSED? The diagnosis is based on the clinical history, risk factors, physical findings and a venous doppler ultrasound of the leg. The ultrasound is able to identify the presence of the clot in the vein. On the scan, it is apparent that the vein is not compressible because it is filled with a blood clot.

WHAT IS THE TREATMENT? The treatment for a DVT involves preventing further development and spread of the clot. Blood thinning agents such as heparin and Coumadin (warfarin) are used. More recently, low molecular weight heparin has been used. A daily dose is injected under the skin for about a week, until the blood is adequately thinned. This can be done at home with proper training.

Coumadin is taken orally and a patient may have to take it for several months. The blood levels are monitored closely so that the blood is adequately thinned, which is called anti-coagulation. If a person is over-anticoagulated, excessive bleeding can occur. Your health care provider will need to monitor this condition slowly and determine the cause for the development of the blood clot.

WHAT ELSE SHOULD I DO? Prevention is the most important aspect of dealing with a DVT. Remaining active during travel is essential. On an airplane, continue to move your legs and get up frequently. If you are in the car, stop frequently, get out and walk around. If you are going to be hospitalized for surgery, your doctors will treat you preventatively. DVTs are generally preventable, so do a few simple things that could save your life. If you feel that you may have a DVT, seek medical attention immediately.

hypertension
(HTN)

It seems like not a day passes when the medical topic of hypertension (high blood pressure) is not discussed in the news media. Hypertension is the root of many health evils and must be taken seriously. Hypertension is a very treatable disease.

WHAT IS HYPERTENSION? Hypertension is an elevation in the blood pressure due to increased forces that are applied against the arteries. The arteries are the blood vessels that carry oxygen-enriched blood away from the heart. When increased force is directed against the blood vessels from the heart, or the vessels have lost their elasticity, the blood pressure will be elevated. This elevation can lead to the development of a variety of medical conditions including coronary artery disease and stroke. These are the two most common problems with the most devastating consequences. Other problems may include peripheral vascular disease, kidney disease, eye disease and congestive heart failure.

WHAT IS AN ELEVATED READING? The standards for blood pressure readings have been extensively studied. In general, a blood pressure reading of 120/80 is considered normal. When blood pressure readings are consistently found between 130-140 and 80-90, there is cause for concern. Consistent readings of blood pressures greater than 140/90 need medical attention.

The pressure is measured by calculating the stress placed against the artery wall and is measured in millimeters of mercury. The top number is the systolic number, which corresponds to the pumping pressure exerted by the heart. The bottom number is the diastolic number and this determines the resting pressure between heartbeats.

WHAT ARE SYMPTOMS OF HYPERTENSION? Hypertension has been referred to as the "silent killer" for years, as there may be no outward signs of the disease besides an elevated blood pressure reading. Of course, long-standing hypertension may cause headaches, nausea and blurred vision, but this is usually not the norm. A person may be first diagnosed during a routine physical. Unfortunately, many people are diagnosed when they suffer their first heart attack or stroke.

BLOOD

WHAT ARE RISK FACTORS FOR DEVELOPING HYPERTEN-SION?

There are a variety of risk factors for the development of hypertension including obesity, lack of exercise, smoking, excessive alcohol or salt intake, and heredity. Many of these risk factors can be modified in order to treat hypertension or prevent its development.

WHAT IS THE TREATMENT? Initially, the risk factors must be modified, including exercise and weight loss. A healthy diet low in salt will be recommended. After these steps have been addressed, a long-term commitment to drug therapy may be necessary.

There are a variety of medications that may be used. Your health care provider will choose which is best based on a variety of factors. Most commonly, a water pill or diuretic may be prescribed. Other medications include beta-blockers, calcium channel blockers and ACE inhibitors, to name just a few. Most of these medications are safe and can be used effectively for a lifetime.

WHAT ELSE SHOULD I DO? As a person ages, it is important to monitor one's blood pressure. Let me caution you about checking your blood pressure too frequently. It is essential that there is consistency in the monitoring process. This means taking the blood pressure in a calm environment by a qualified evaluator with reasonable equipment.

In the emergency department, a day does not usually pass when someone arrives because they are alarmed by the elevated reading of the local store's free blood pressure monitor. This is usually an isolated reading that does not mandate treatment. Elevated blood pressure readings do not require immediate treatment. Cases that need immediate intervention in the hospital are quite rare.

Most importantly, the diagnosis of hypertension must be made over a period of time. Then, lifestyles must be changed prior to instituting a lifetime of costly medications. It is essential that close medical follow up and management be initiated when there are risks for hypertension. Start by obtaining a baseline reading and seeking medical counseling when you are at risk. You may be able to prevent a medical catastrophe.

pulmonary embolism

As the events of the Iraqi war unfold, we have been exposed to many losses, including that of NBC reporter David Bloom. At the age of 39, Bloom succumbed to a pulmonary embolism, a blood clot that had developed in his body. There were symptoms, but unaware of what was traveling through his system, Bloom ignored those signs and kept on working full throttle at his job. Could this have been prevented? Could he have been saved?

WHAT IS A PULMONARY EMBOLISM? An embolism is a blood clot that travels from one part of the body to another causing problems. This type of blood clot usually travels from the larger vessels of the lower body and extremities into the lungs. Blocking circulation in the lungs, the clot prevents further oxygenation of the blood. A whole cascade of events occurs, but the patient essentially dies from lack of oxygen.

HOW COMMON IS A PULMONARY EMBOLISM? In the United States, there are hundreds of millions of pulmonary embolism cases diagnosed each year. Of those cases, over 200,000 Americans die annually and it is responsible for 15 percent of all in-hospital deaths. Pulmonary embolism is the third leading cause of death in this country!

HOW DOES IT DEVELOP? As we all know, it is normal for the blood to clot when it is outside our body. The problem occurs when the blood clots inside the blood vessels. The most common blood clots found traveling to the lungs usually come from the legs. These clots are referred to as deep venous thrombosis or DVTs.

The development of clots in the vessels may be caused by several events including inactivity or sitting for long periods of time in cramped quarters. An example of this is "economy class syndrome," a term arising from sitting in an airplane on a long flight without moving. The blood tends to pool in the legs and eventually clots. Once the clotting cascade starts, it can be difficult to stop. These clots eventually break into pieces traveling elsewhere in the body causing a life-threatening emergency.

BLOOD

ARE THERE OTHER CAUSES? Yes. The risk factors for the development of blood clots include prolonged immobilization. Other factors that place a patient at risk for a pulmonary embolism include recent surgery, severe burns, trauma, pregnancy or post-partum, obesity, cancer, heart disease and blood disease.

WHAT ARE THE SYMPTOMS? There are a wide variety of nonspecific symptoms, which make the diagnosis very, very difficult. The most common symptoms include shortness of breath, chest wall pain, rapid heart rate, weakness, coughing up blood, anxiety or calf swelling. Unfortunately for some people, there are no warning signs and sudden collapse with death occurs. It is apparent that a pulmonary embolism mimics many conditions, and is therefore referred to as the "Great Masquerader."

HOW IS IT DIAGNOSED? Making the diagnosis is difficult. The health care provider must take a very accurate and detailed history and complete a physical examination. The provider must have a clinical suspicion that the patient is at risk.

Then, the pieces of the puzzle will need to be assembled. Blood testing may help, but may not be definitive. x-ray studies will include a chest x-ray, possibly a nuclear medicine procedure called a lung scan, and possibly a CT scan of the chest. The most invasive procedure may involve angiography, whereby a physician will inject dye into the vessels of the lungs and complete additional x-ray pictures. Additional testing may include an ultrasound (sound wave picture) of the vessels of the legs.

WHAT IS THE TREATMENT? In the event that a patient experiences a pulmonary embolism, they will possibly receive a clot-busting drug, called a fibrinolytic, that is given in the vein. The patient will also be placed on heparin, a blood-thinning drug. Long-term therapy will necessitate the patient to taking warfarin (Coumadin), an oral blood-thinning drug. All of this will be completed during a hospitalization.

WHAT SHOULD I DO? In the event that you experience any of the above-described symptoms with associated risk factors, you must seek medical attention immediately. Call 911. Death can occur very quickly, just as it did with David Bloom.

You can protect yourself by taking an aspirin daily, but this should be at the direction of your health care provider. Aspirin is a wonderful medication, but not without side effects. Additionally, if you are on a long trip, take time to exercise and move your legs. Drink fluids, as dehydration may contribute to blood clot development. As always, in the event that you have concerns, seek medical attention by a qualified provider. You may be saving your own life!

stasis ulcer

We seem to spend a great deal of time discussing ulcers that are associated with the gastrointestinal system. Yet, there is another type of ulcer that develops on the lower legs and feet, unrelated to the gastrointestinal system. They usually affect older individuals and may be quite chronic in nature.

WHAT IS A STASIS ULCER? This skin condition occurs in an area of sluggish blood flow, most commonly around the ankle. The pooling of blood in the lower extremity is caused by "poor circulation". This leads to skin break-down and the development of an ulcer that looks like a crater.

Stasis comes from the Greek derivative meaning the posture of standing. These ulcers are usually chronic, meaning that they last a long time and are very difficult to heal. Once the skin breaks down, there may be swelling, inflammation and infection in the area. This makes treatment and resolution much more difficult.

ARE THERE DIFFERENT TYPES OF ULCERS? Yes. There are three different types of ulcers that are related to vascular supply. The most common ulcer is the venous stasis ulcer that is due to the backup of blood in the legs, secondary to bad veins. Most commonly, varicose veins are the culprits.

With varicose veins, the return of the blood back up the leg toward the heart is impaired. This leads to pooling of blood in the legs and swelling. There may also be a fluid overload due to a bad heart, which is called congestive heart failure. All of this increased stress on the legs stretches and damages the skin. When this happens, the skin is much more fragile. About a half million Americans are affected by these types of ulcers.

Less common types of ulcers are arterial ulcers. This is due to very poor, oxygen-rich, arterial blood supply. Patients that have peripheral vascular disease due to smoking, high cholesterol or hereditary factors may develop these ulcers. These ulcers are differentiated from other ulcers due to lack of bleeding and extreme pain.

BLOOD

Lastly, diabetics can develop ulcers in the lower extremity due to a combination of factors. They may develop peripheral neuropathy, which are damaged nerves due to diabetes. With the loss of sensation in the legs and feet, a diabetic may not realize that they have been injured. For example, a stone in a shoe will not be felt, and after a full day of walking, a blister will develop. Due to poor circulation and diabetic skin changes, an ulcer will develop. This can be very difficult to treat and also recurrent.

WHAT ARE THE CAUSES? Poor circulation and blood supply is the leading cause for the development of lower extremity ulcers. Increased vascular pressure or lack of good blood supply will change the texture of the skin. It will become thinned and fragile. When this occurs, it will not easily heal once injured. The skin may change in color due to the chronic damage. An infection may be present and pus may drain from the wound. If the condition gets out of control, the infection may seep into other parts of the body leading to sepsis and death.

WHAT IS THE TREATMENT? The diagnosis is made by clinical history and appearance of the wound. Local immediate treatment may include treating the infection and stopping the offending factors. Your health care provider will need to help improve circulation and prevent swelling in the lower extremity. Heart conditions must be addressed as well.

As a patient, smoking cessation is essential in order to help improve blood flow. Diabetics must have tight control of their blood sugars, as diabetes inhibits healing. Daily trips to a wound clinic might be necessary to heal the ulcer.

Prevention is essential, and once healed, the vascular system must be assessed. Surgery may even be necessary to improve circulation. Your health care provider may require you to wear elastic stockings. Most importantly, if you develop this condition, seek immediate medical attention, as this condition will not usually heal itself.

varicose veins

Remember the terrible sausage-like veins on your grandmother's legs? She would wear heavy stockings and complain a lot about the pain in her legs. As a child, you were convinced that you would never have such terrible looking legs. But, time has caught up with you and now your legs look very similar. Fortunately, you have more options, both medical and surgical, to deal with varicose veins than your grandmother did.

WHAT ARE VARICOSE VEINS? Varicose veins are swollen stretched out veins that are engorged in blood. Most varicose veins are found in the legs and this article will focus on those varicosities. Varicose veins can be found elsewhere in the body and another type of varicose vein is a hemorrhoid. This topic will be dealt with in a later chapter.

HOW DO VARICOSE VEINS FORM? In the lower extremity, blood is returned "uphill" by the veins. In order to prevent backflow of the blood, veins have valves. These valves act as a one-way dam. When these valves become weakened, they allow the blood to flow backward. This backflow of blood leads to damming up of the blood and the veins become swollen and congested.

WHY DO THEY FORM? There are a variety of reasons that varicose veins form. Humans may have a hereditary factor that contributes to their formation. The veins may be predisposed to having weakened valves. This, in combination with repetitive trauma, such as prolonged standing, may contribute to their formation. In addition, other factors include obesity, aging, hormones and pregnancy.

HOW COMMON ARE VARICOSE VEINS? They are fairly common and up to 60 percent of all Americans will develop a form of a varicose vein. Up to 50 percent of all women will develop varicosities some time in their life, and 41 percent of all women will have varicose veins by the age of 50.

BLOOD

HOW CAN I PREVENT VARICOSE VEINS? You cannot change your genetics, but you can do a few simple things to help prevent the development of varicose veins. Exercise is important in helping develop excellent circulation and vein strength. Obesity is a major risk factor, so weight control and reduction are essential. Do not sit with the legs crossed, as this blocks return circulation, damaging the valves of the veins.

A job that requires standing for prolonged periods of time significantly contributes to the weakening of the valves in the veins. If you must stand for a long time, shift weight from leg to leg. Also, it is important to wear support stockings, but be careful that they are not too tight.

WHAT MEDICAL AND SURGICAL TREATMENTS ARE AVAILABLE? Once varicose veins have developed and become unsightly and painful, a trip to the doctor's office may be necessary. You may need to see a vascular surgeon or a specialist that deals with varicose veins.

Medical and surgical treatment may include the use of chemicals to dry up the veins, called sclerotherapy. The process involves injecting a chemical into the vein that will cause the vein to swell and eventually close it off. The vein becomes scarred and the circulation will be routed around this vein. This is generally not a problem, as the body develops additional blood supply called collateral circulation.

Recent treatments also include the use of electricity and lasers to burn the vein, causing them to close. Some of these procedures are new and must be discussed with your doctor.

The old standby treatment has included the surgical removal of the large damaged veins. This procedure is very effective, but may require hospitalization and a prolonged period of rehabilitation.

WHAT ELSE CAN I DO? As always, prevention is the best treatment. Take the time to exercise and be healthy. This will improve your chances of not being affected. In the event that you need medical and surgical treatment, be sure to find a specialist that is well versed in a variety of treatment options and has a proven record of successfully treated and satisfied patients.

adult attention deficit disorder
(ADD)

Do you have trouble concentrating on just one thing or start multiple projects and then not finish them? Have trouble organizing yourself? Do you procrastinate when a project requires attention to detail? Have trouble remembering appointments? Are you fidgety? Lose a lot of things?

Perhaps I just described your life or that of someone you know. Granted, we all experience many of these characteristics some time in our lives, but there are those of us who are plagued with these qualities on a daily basis. This may make someone miserable and they may be called a variety of names such as "scatterbrains" or "clueless", but they may indeed have a treatable medical condition.

WHAT IS THIS CONDITION? There has been a lot of publicity concerning this disorder called Adult Attention Deficit Disorder (ADD) or Adult Attention Deficit Hyperactivity Disorder (ADHD). In general, Adult ADD is the more common term, as the hyperactivity component of this disorder usually fades in adulthood.

HOW COMMON IS THIS CONDITION? Adult ADD is a fairly common condition affecting about 4 percent of all adults. It is certainly more common in children with 6-9 percent prevalence. It is interesting to see that in the 1970s, ADD was thought to only affect children and that the disorder was outgrown. What has happened is that some children gain better control of their symptoms and the hyperactivity component seems to diminish in adulthood. It is clear that the impulsive acts may persist throughout an adult life.

WHAT ARE THE SYMPTOMS? Medical professionals have identified some key symptoms that may be suggestive of Adult ADD. These include difficulty in paying attention, easily distracted, difficulty planning and meeting deadlines, interrupting others while speaking, difficulty following directions, procrastination and impulsivity.

Many of these symptoms may be present and persistent. Periods of stress can make it difficult for the person to perform. A great deal of individuals with Adult ADD are very creative and energetic. When appropriately directed,

BRAIN

they can accomplish a lot of things. Unfortunately, this condition can interfere with interpersonal relationships at home, school and work.

WHAT CAN BE DONE? Initially, one must be suspect of the disorder. Today, it seems that we are much more in tune to the disorder and better able to consider ADD as a diagnosis. There are several simple screening tools that are available from your health care provider or even on the Internet. The screening tool may include a self-assessment questionnaire. Once there is suspicion that an adult may suffer from ADD, professional help should be sought.

WHAT IS THE TREATMENT? After a firm diagnosis is made by a health care professional, a variety of treatment options may be proposed depending on the severity of the disorder, as well as other associated conditions such as depression or anxiety.

Initial treatment may include a variety of behavior modification techniques and recommendations to become organized and stay organized. A simple modification may include the use of checklists and reminders that will help the individual keep focused.

The use of medication has long proven successful in children and the use of stimulants such as Ritalin and Adderall have been used. It may seem confusing that physicians would prescribe a stimulant to a hyperactive person, but it has what is called a paradoxical (opposite) effect. A new medication was approved in January 2003, called Strattera, which does have an indication for Adult ADD. The success of this medication still needs to be evaluated.

WHAT SHOULD I DO? If you believe that you or a friend suffers from Adult ADD, you need to gather some information. The Internet is a very powerful information tool, but you must be careful. I recommend websites that are sponsored by an academic institution, such as a medical school.

If you feel that the diagnosis of Adult ADD applies to your situation, seek a health professional that is well versed in the subject and treatment. A recent study has shown that only a third of physicians that provide primary care are knowledgeable in the treatment of the disorder. A wide variety of treatments are available that offer hope for a full and enriching life.

alzheimer's disease

DOES THIS SOUND FAMILIAR TO YOU?

"Mom, how are you today?"
"Good honey. Where's your dad?"
"Dad's been gone for some time Mom."
"Oh yeah, well when's your aunt coming to visit me?"
"Mom, your sister's gone, too."
"Who are you?"
"Mom it's me, your daughter."
"Good to see you again, it's been so long."
"I was just here yesterday, Mom. But it's good to see you again, too."

Unfortunately, this conversation is all too common and something I've seen frequently in my 15 years practicing emergency medicine.

Emergency departments across the United States are filled with elderly patients who have complex medical problems, many which require hospitalization and comprehensive therapy. Along with this aging population, comes another disease process, Alzheimer's disease (AD).

Over 4.5 million Americans currently suffer from AD and this number will grow to 16 million by the year 2050. A recent study has shown the relationship between diabetes and the progression of AD. Diabetics face a 65 percent higher chance of developing Alzheimer's. Unfortunately, there is no cure for the disease, but the research continues.

WHAT IS ALZHEIMER'S DISEASE? AD is a progressive neurologic disease that affects the brain and is universally fatal. The brain begins to degenerate and there is loss of memory, impaired thinking, diminished cognition and unusual behavior. Changes in behavior range from depression to agitation. This is the most common form of dementia seen in patients over the age of 65. It is very unusual to see this problem in younger folks. Once diagnosed, the average lifespan with the disease is 8 years.

AD is named after the German physician, Alois Alzheimer, who first discovered the process in 1906. It was once a rare problem, but is now considered a major health care issue among the elderly.

BRAIN

WHAT ARE THE RISKS AND CAUSES? There is no known cause for AD, but it is known that the number one risk factor is progression of age. Each person with AD is affected differently and it is difficult to predict how each person will respond and progress throughout the illness.

It is known that AD has a genetic predisposition and it does run in families. There is an early form of AD that can be present between the ages of 30 to 60 years and this has a definite genetic origin. The more common type of AD that presents after the age of 65 has less genetic prevalence. Some studies have shown a protein link in the blood of patients, but more research is required to further identify this link.

HOW IS IT DIAGNOSED? There is no specific test that can aid the health care provider with an easy diagnosis. As with most conditions, a comprehensive history must be taken, followed by a physical examination. A battery of baseline laboratory studies will be run and a CT scan of the brain will be completed. All of this is done to rule out any other reversible metabolic or medical conditions. A primary care provider will complete a great deal of the initial work up and then a neurologist (brain specialist) may be consulted. Next, a variety of mental function tests will be performed to confirm the diagnosis.

WHAT ARE THE WARNING SIGNS OF AD? The Alzheimer's Association has identified ten warning signs of AD. These signs include memory loss and difficulty in performing simple familiar tasks. There may be problems with language and word finding. Eventually, a person may have trouble with orientation to time and place. There may be changes in judgment and abstract thinking. Later on, there may be changes in mood, personality and behavior. Lastly, one may see a change in motivation and initiative with regard to activities of daily life. Ultimately, if you begin to observe any of these warning signs in those that are close to you, it would be wise to pursue an evaluation.

WHAT IS THE TREATMENT? At the present time, there is no cure for AD. There are certain medications that have been used to slow the progression of the disease or stabilize it. They work on certain brain chemicals and many patients have responded favorably to these medications.

Once the diagnosis is made, it is essential to involve the patient and the family in planning for the future. Advanced directives should be in place to help with end-of-life decisions during times of crisis. Early disclosure to family and friends is important in allowing everyone to gain an understanding of the process.

In time, families and patients may need to made decisions for additional care arrangements at an appropriate facility. This a very stressful situation for family members and they, too, will need support during this time.

For more information on AD, or resources for living with AD, visit the Alzheimer's Association website at www.alz.org. This website will provide you with information on the nationwide network of more than 80 support groups and 220 local points of service.

aneurysm

The wife of Senator John McCain of Arizona suffered the rupture of a cerebral aneurysm. This is where a blood vessel in the brain bursts and leaks blood. Recent reports have been positive for Cindy McCain, as she was released from the hospital after four days of treatment. She suffered a small stroke that affected her speech, but she apparently has very little residual. Apparently, she stopped taking her blood pressure medicine and this was the cause for the stroke. Elevations in blood pressure can cause a cerebral aneurysm to rupture, so let's look a little more closely at cerebral aneurysms.

WHAT IS A CEREBRAL ANEURYSM? An aneurysm is any weakening and dilation of a blood vessel. This can occur primarily in any artery of the body, but the most common area of aneurysms is in the brain. These aneurysms affect the arteries that supply the brain and can become weakened from a variety of stresses on the vessel. The dilation looks like a little balloon that occurs in a weakened area of a water hose.

HOW COMMON ARE CEREBRAL ANEURYSMS? Medical studies have shown that about 3 to 6 percent of all Americans have a cerebral aneurysm and most are asymptomatic. The diagnosis is made in a majority of the cases once the blood vessel ruptures and other symptoms are present. It has also been shown that the larger the aneurysm, the greater the chance of rupture.

Studies have shown that aneurysms less that 10 millimeters (mm) have a small chance of rupture, 10 to 20 mm have a greater chance and those over 25 mm have a very significant chance of rupture. Therefore, the latter two require more aggressive evaluation and treatment such as surgical repair.

WHAT ARE THE RISK FACTORS FOR DEVELOPING AN ANEURYSM? High blood pressure is one of the most common risks for developing this problem. In addition, it has been shown that smoking, age over 50 years, cocaine use, female gender, trauma, and tumors are contributing factors. There are a variety of hereditary medical conditions that affect blood vessel walls such as polycystic kidney disease and conditions affecting the elastin in the body. The hereditary diseases are rare. It should be remembered that there is increased risk if two or more family members have had a cerebral aneurysm.

BRAIN

WHAT ARE THE SYMPTOMS? Most clinical presentations of an aneurysm are associated with a leakage or rupture of the blood vessel. Acutely, a person may complain of the worst headache of their life. There may be a change in mental status, vision, paralysis, or unconsciousness. Nearly two thirds of all patients have this late presentation with significant symptoms.

If there is suspicion of an aneurysm, it may be found incidentally on a screening exam. Screening exams are only worthwhile in persons with significant risk factors such as a strong family history of aneurysms, specific hereditary conditions, prolonged untreated hypertension, and some neurological complaints of headache and blurred vision. In general, these incidental discoveries are rare.

HOW IS IT DIAGNOSED? As with most conditions, clinical suspicion is important. Based on the risk factors, a CT scan or MRI scan of the brain may be completed. Currently, MRI angiography, which fills the blood vessels with a dye during the x-ray, is a very common procedure. If the initial x-ray study is negative, a spinal tap may be performed to check for the presence of blood in the cerebral spinal fluid, which would indicate that the vessel is leaking.

WHAT IS THE TREATMENT? There are varied opinions on treatment. The unruptured small aneurysm does not require intervention. Monitoring of the size and blood pressure is essential. The larger aneurysms of greater than 10 mm may require surgical correction. Unfortunately, surgical correction is not without complications. Your health care provider must outline the risks, benefits, and alternatives to the condition, as the pros and cons must be closely evaluated. Complications from surgery can include a stroke, paralysis, altered mental status and death.

WHAT ELSE SHOULD I DO? Monitoring and treating high blood pressure is an excellent preventative measure, as well as quitting smoking. Random screenings are of little benefit, as each case must be evaluated for risk factors and potential symptoms. Additionally, seeking medical advice if concerned is essential, as this may prevent a lifetime of disability.

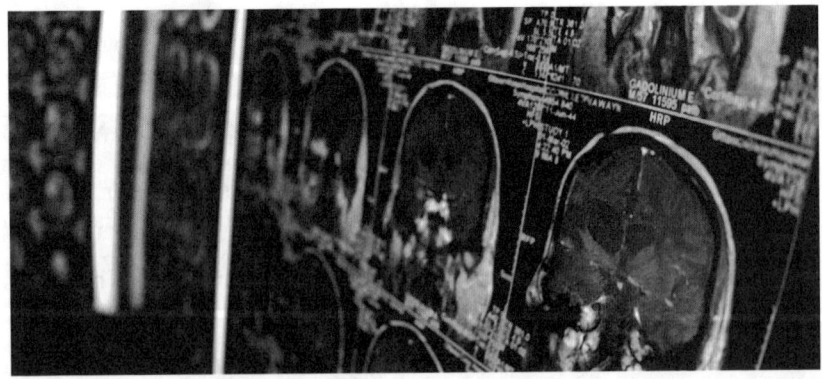

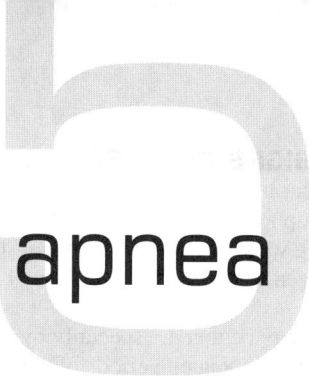

apnea

The death of former Green Bay Packer, Reggie White, heightened our awareness of a fairly common medical condition known as sleep apnea. Over the past several years, more information about this condition has become available, as well as diagnostic testing and treatment. It is thought that White suffered a deadly heart rhythm that was caused by his sleep apnea.

WHAT IS SLEEP APNEA? The term apnea comes from the Greek phrase meaning "without breath or want to breathe." This means that a person actually stops breathing while they sleep. Apnea, by definition, means lack of a breath for 10 or more seconds. These involuntary events can usually range from 20 to 60 times per hour, which is quite significant.

IS THIS A COMMON PROBLEM? Yes. It has been shown that between 12 to 18 million Americans suffer from this condition at a variety of levels. Obviously, White's level of sleep apnea was quite severe, which lead to his untimely death.

There are two types of sleep apnea– central sleep apnea and obstructive sleep apnea. The central form is quite rare and caused by a brain abnormality that does not tell the body to breathe. Obstructive sleep apnea is the most common form, which does not allow for adequate passage of air during the sleep cycle.

WHAT ARE THE CAUSES? The causes of sleep apnea are numerous and can usually be corrected. During the normal sleep cycle, the muscles and soft tissues of the upper airway relax, thereby blocking the passage of air. Individuals with a normal sleep cycle have a large enough airway that will allow air and oxygen to pass, even in the very relaxed state. When the body is depleted of adequate oxygen, the brain will stimulate the body to wake up, opening the airway and allowing for a breath.

Risk factors for obstructive sleep apnea include obesity, structural facial abnormalities, snoring and excessive use of alcohol. Some other medical conditions can contribute to this problem as well.

BRAIN

WHAT ARE THE SIGNS OF SLEEP APNEA? A clinician may be suspicious that a patient has sleep apnea when the patient complains of problems such as waking up not feeling rested, waking up numerous times during the night and suffering with a morning headache. The headache may be due to a chronic lack of oxygen.

Other symptoms that may be noted, especially by a spouse of an affected patient, include snoring, associated periods of apnea, excessive daytime sleepiness, weight gain, lack of attention, memory loss and personality changes. Many times, it is the concern of the spouse that brings the patient to the doctor. About the same number of men and women are affected, but more men than women are diagnosed.

HOW IS THIS DIAGNOSED? A health care provider must be suspect when a patient presents with complaints of a sleep disorder. This should be followed by a comprehensive physical examination. Blood testing may show lack of oxygen.

Physical abnormalities in the jaw, mouth, and face should be identified. Snoring is a hallmark for sleep apnea, indicating a structural abnormality in the upper airway.

The next step may include a sleep study, conducted by a physician specializing in sleep disorders. The sleep study involves monitoring a patient during sleep. Vital signs, oxygen content, and heart rhythm are recorded during an entire sleep cycle. When completed, the data is collected and analyzed.

WHAT IS THE TREATMENT? Once identified, a patient may need to undergo weight reduction, which may cure the problem. The other most commonly recommended treatment is the use of the continuous positive airway pressure (CPAP) mask, which is worn at night. This device fits snugly over the nose or mouth and nose, actually forcing oxygen in and keeping the airway open.

In the event of structural abnormalities, jaw devices or surgery may be necessary. A surgery to correct snoring is another way to deal with the problem. The surgery may remove some tissue in the back of the throat making the airway larger and not allowing it to collapse during a relaxed state. Lastly, it is important that the use of alcohol be controlled, as this may be a factor contributing to the problem.

depression

Throughout life, everyone experiences events that are upsetting and make one feel sad. These feelings may be disruptive and last for a few days. It is completely normal to experience these feelings of depression when related to a certain event. When these symptoms persist for weeks or months, a problem has developed and this medical issue must be addressed. Depression is a medical condition that can be cured with appropriate psychological and medical treatment.

WHAT IS DEPRESSION? Depression is a mood disorder whereby one feels sad or blue. When these feelings persist continuously over a two week period, a diagnosis of clinical depression is in order. There are several forms of depression that each have their own characteristic features.

WHAT ARE SOME CHARACTERISTIC FEATURES? In order to make a diagnosis of major depression, at least five of the following symptoms must be present. One must have a depressed mood for the majority of the day. There is no ability to find pleasure in life's activities. There are problems with sleep, including insomnia or excessive sleep. There may be a change in appetite with weight change. There may be agitation or lethargy. A person may feel guilty or worthless. The person may also have difficulty concentrating. Finally, one may be suicidal.

WHAT ARE OTHER DEPRESSIVE CONDITIONS? About 6 percent of Americans suffer from dysthymia or chronic depression. A patient with dysthymia may have many of the features of a major depressive condition, but the symptoms are less intense and last longer. Patients experiencing dysthymia have a veil of sadness and have difficulty enjoying any aspect of daily life. A sense of negativism seems to prevail in their lives.

During the winter months, many people suffer from Seasonal Affective Disorder (SAD). It seems that lack of sunshine and inclement weather are inciting factors and may last for up to five months, especially in people living in the northern United States. SAD is characterized by oversleeping, over-eating and a generalized sense of fatigue and lethargy.

BRAIN

WHAT CAUSES DEPRESSION? It is known that depression tends to run in families, so there is a genetic predisposition to the development of depression.

Alterations in brain chemicals such as serotonin, dopamine, epinephrine and norepinephrine have been shown to be a causive factor. It has been specifically shown that an alteration in the regulation of serotonin by the brain can lead to depression.

It is also known that changes in hormones can lead to a depressive state. In addition, it is interesting to note some patients who suffer from depression actually have alterations in their brain structure. Another interesting fact is that people with insomnia have a 20 percent chance of developing depression and 90 percent of all depressed people suffer from insomnia!

HOW IS DEPRESSION DIAGNOSED? Your health care provider must make the diagnosis based on a comprehensive history and physical examination. There are many questionnaires that can help the clinician make the diagnosis. After any medical conditions are ruled out, treatment may ensue.

HOW IS IT TREATED? There are a variety of treatments available for depression. Psychological counseling is usually encouraged and is very effective. This may involve the patient and family members.

Depending on the magnitude of the state of depression, a variety of medicines are available. Most commonly, clinicians prescribe the Selective Serotonin Reuptake Inhibitors (SSRI's) quite safely and effectively. If these do not work, there are a variety of other safe anti-depressants available.

More severe cases of depression that have not responded to medical therapy may require hospitalization, especially if the patient is at risk for harming himself or herself. A health care professional must evaluate for suicidal thoughts and gestures. Lastly, electroconvulsive therapy (ECT), which is electrical brain stimulation, has a proven success rate. A psychiatrist, who is proficient in this procedure, must administer this.

WHAT SHOULD I DO? If you or someone you know appears depressed, seek medical attention. Depression is the second most common diagnosis in the family physician's office, with high blood pressure leading the list. Depression is a medical condition that can be effectively and safely treated with medication and psychological therapy.

To Your Health with Dr. Wojo

dizziness

Dizziness is a frequent complaint in the ER and at the doctor's office. In fact, it's so common that it accounts for over eight million doctor visits in the United States each year!

Dizziness is a term that is actually used to describe several different types of feelings, like the sensation of spinning, unsteadiness or wooziness. Rapid head movements can make the sensation worse.

Dizziness may come on very quickly, and unfortunately recovery may be slow. Sometimes it takes several days — or even several weeks — before the patient returns to feeling normal again.

WHAT CAUSES DIZZINESS? Dizziness is not actually a disease, but a symptom indicating a problem with the balance mechanism of the inner ear, or a disturbance within the brain. Medical conditions that can contribute to dizziness include high blood pressure, diabetes, heart disease or a prior infection or neurological disease (such as a stroke). Don't let this scare you, though. Most conditions are not life threatening, and there are usually no real major physical problems, but dizziness does call for a visit to your doctor.

Are there different "types" of dizziness? There are actually four major categories of dizziness: vertigo, presyncope, dysequilibrium and light-headedness.

Vertigo is a sense of false motion between a person and the outside world. Many patients usually describe a feeling that the room is spinning. There may also be some nausea, vomiting, paleness and sweating. There is no loss of consciousness or headache, but it sometimes comes on very quickly and many times occurs in the middle of the night, requiring a visit to the ER.

Presyncope is a feeling that a person is about to faint. Patients sometimes describe buzzing in the ears, rubbery legs, changes in vision, sweating and nausea. This is usually caused by lack of blood supply to the brain, which can occur when someone stands in one position for too long. It can be a one-time or recurring problem.

BRAIN

Dysequilibrium is the feeling that someone is going to lose their balance or pass out, and it usually occurs while standing or walking. It often happens as people get older and the body loses its ability to quickly adjust to changes in position or terrain. However, when a young patient has these symptoms, there is concern that there may be a neurological problem.

Light-headedness is a very vague sensation that is not well-defined. In fact, the condition is usually so mild that the patient can't describe the exact feeling to the doctor. It may be only caused by anxiety or hyperventilation, but doctors are always careful not to rule out any larger problems when patients complain of light-headedness.

HOW IS MY PROBLEM DIAGNOSED? When visiting the doctor's office or ER because of dizziness, the most important tool in helping a doctor reach a diagnosis is a detailed and accurate history of the symptoms. The doctor will ask many questions to figure out exactly what sensations the patient is experiencing. Some doctors may even have their patients fill out a questionnaire.

Usually, diagnostic testing is not required with simple cases of dizziness. However, in severe cases, x-ray imaging of the brain, like Computerized Axial Tomography (CT scan) or Magnetic Resonance Imaging (MRI), may be needed to look for any structural problems in the brain.

HOW IS IT TREATED? After a diagnosis is made, a doctor may prescribe medications that work by stabilizing structures within the inner ear and brain responsible for dizziness. Some doctors have even been successful in treating dizziness with head motions called the Pike-Hall maneuvers — these are therapeutic head turning movements that your physician may prescribe to help reset the balance mechanism.

Remember, most cases of dizziness are not caused by serious physical problems, but you should see your doctor just to be sure.

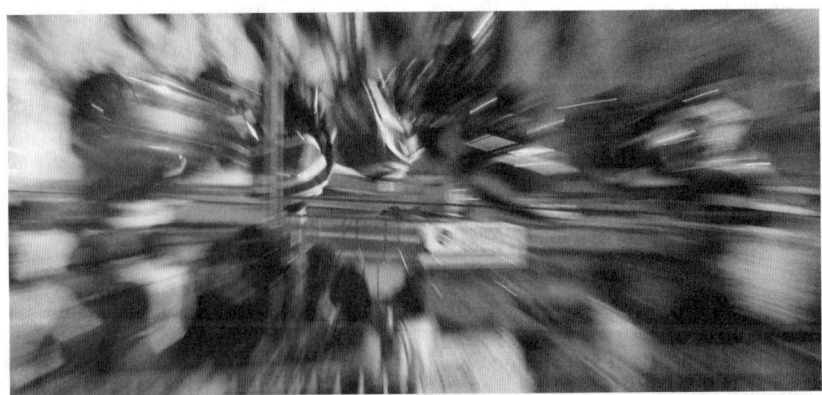

To Your Health with Dr. Wojo

excessive daytime sleepiness (EDS)

The Federal Drug Administration recently added a clinical indication for a drug that was approved in 2002 for the treatment of narcolepsy, which is the brain's inability to maintain proper sleep cycles. The medicine, Xyrem, is a formulation of Gamma Hydroxybutyrate, and has specific indications for the treatment of narcolepsy, a serious sleep disorder. The most recent FDA drug indication is for the treatment of Excessive Daytime Sleepiness (EDS).

WHAT IS EDS? This problem is a sleep disorder where an individual has the uncontrolled urge to fall asleep in the middle of the day. The problem is not related to lack of sleep from staying up too late watching TV, partying too long, or working shift work. This problem occurs in very well-rested individuals who just cannot stay awake in the middle of the day. This is also referred to as somnolence or hypersomnia.

EDS is not usually caused by lack of sleep or sleep deprivation. There may be some medical causes that can lead to this problem. The causes may include a brain injury or tumor that has disrupted the nervous system. There may be other associated sleep problems such as sleep apnea or narcolepsy. Certain medications can interrupt sleep patterns. Drug and alcohol abuse may also contribute to alterations in sleep and waking cycles.

There are some medical problems that interfere with sleep, and they include multiple sclerosis, infection, depression and obesity. All of these conditions may contribute to the development of a sleep disorder that ultimately may lead to EDS.

WHAT ARE THE SYMPTOMS OF EDS? There are wide ranges of symptoms that can be nonspecific to EDS. These symptoms may include constant fatigue, lethargy, lack of concentration and irritability. The patient may sleep excessively for 10-12 hours per night and then will require a couple daytime naps. Many of these people are perceived as lazy. This truly is not the case.

BRAIN

HOW IS THIS DIAGNOSED? When a patient sleeps poorly for a month or longer, an evaluation is necessary. Initially, a workup by a primary health care provider will include a history and physical examination. Some blood work may be necessary to rule out any medical problem. If nothing is found, a referral to a sleep specialist is in order. This is usually a neurologist with specialized training in sleep disorders.

The next step will be a sleep study to assess the quality of sleep. Sleep apnea may be diagnosed during this process. An individual will go to a sleep lab and be closely monitored for a night. Naps may be evaluated, as well as periods of wakefulness.

WHAT IS THE TREATMENT? A wide variety of treatments may be recommended, depending on the cause of the problem. Good sleep hygiene will be recommended, which includes simple things to prepare for bedtime. Avoidance of alcohol and certain medications may be in order as well. If sleep apnea is an issue, a CPAP mask may be prescribed to help keep open the airway during sleep, along with providing supplemental oxygen.

Xyrem may be used to help improve stages 3 and 4 of sleep. Improved sleep at this time will lead to fewer complications during the day. This medication is highly controlled and can only be administered by doctors approved to do so. It is very costly and in the range of over $600 per month. The use of this medication has potential for abuse, so the patient must be closely monitored.

Sleep issues are very complex and complicated. The resolution to the problem is not always easy. Most importantly, if you or a family member suffers from a significant sleep disorder, seek medical attention from a qualified specialist. Several treatment options are available that may change a life.

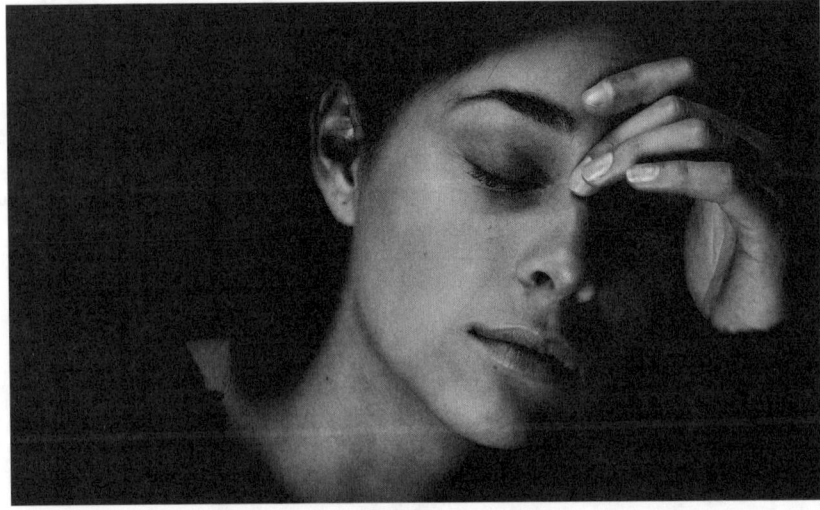

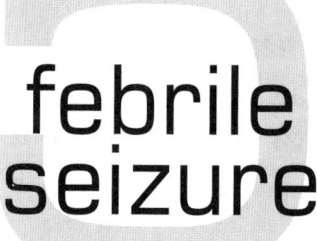

febrile seizure

There is nothing scarier than to be having a quiet evening with your family, and all of a sudden, a child starts to have a seizure. This situation can just pop up out of nowhere and you need to react. The appearance of your child having a seizure is unnerving and so unexpected. Does this mean a lifetime of seizures? Probably not. You take your child's temperature and it is 102°F. Your child has just had a febrile seizure.

WHAT IS A FEBRILE SEIZURE? A febrile seizure is a convulsion that is brought on by a sudden elevation in temperature, usually 102° F or higher. The convulsion is when the child loses consciousness and begins to flail around with jerking movements of the arms and legs. This may last for a few seconds or a few minutes. The electrical system of the brain has gotten out of control and discharged itself. Once it is over, the electrical system of the brain needs to recover and the child may be confused or sleepy. This resolves in several minutes.

IS THIS A COMMON PROBLEM? Yes. About 2 to 4 percent of American children will experience one febrile seizure by the age of 5. Seizures may start around six months of age and rarely occur over the age of 5. As the name implies, the condition is brought on by a fever and does not usually mean that your child has epilepsy. Less than 2 percent of children with febrile seizures go on to develop a seizure disorder. Most of these cases will resolve with increased age.

DO THEY REOCCUR? Yes. Children who experience febrile seizures are at risk for having more seizures when they develop a temperature. Some children are just more prone to these seizures and a family history of other children having febrile seizures puts siblings at risk.

DO FEBRILE SEIZURES HARM A CHILD? In general, there is no risk to a child that has a febrile seizure. There are risks of children hurting themselves when they have a seizure due to falling down and striking something. But, the child is not at risk for brain damage from the seizure or the fever. Of course, if there is a serious underlying medical problem such as meningitis, brain damage can occur. It is essential for the health care provider to determine if this is the case through further testing.

BRAIN

WHAT IS THE TREATMENT? For parents, it is important to remain calm and protect the child from further injury such as falling off a bed or striking a solid object. The child should be placed on their side if possible to help keep the airway clear. Never place anything in the mouth to try and keep it open, as the object may be swallowed. It will seem like the seizure is lasting a long time, but usually it will stop within a few seconds to a couple of minutes. If your child continues to have seizures, then it is important to call 911 and summon emergency medical assistance. The child will be taken in for further medical evaluation.

WHAT IS DONE AT THE HOSPITAL? If the seizure is determined to be from a fever, a source for the temperature elevation will be pursued. Fevers may be secondary to viral infections and bacterial infections. Bacterial infections will require antibiotics to treat the infection. Most commonly, the source may be the ears, throat, lungs or urine. Usually, if a child has an infection of the fluid around the brain, which is meningitis, the child will be quite ill and the seizures may not stop. This is a fairly uncommon occurrence.

WHAT ELSE IS DONE? Most importantly, the source of the fever must be identified and then the fever is treated. The most effective treatment is through the use of acetaminophen (Tylenol) and ibuprofen (Motrin, Advil). It is very important to pay attention to scheduled dosing of these medications. There are some children that do have a seizure with every fever and they may require the use of the sedative Valium to prevent the seizures from occurring. Most importantly, remember that this is not a serious, life-threatening condition, so remain calm and protect your child. Then, seek appropriate medical attention.

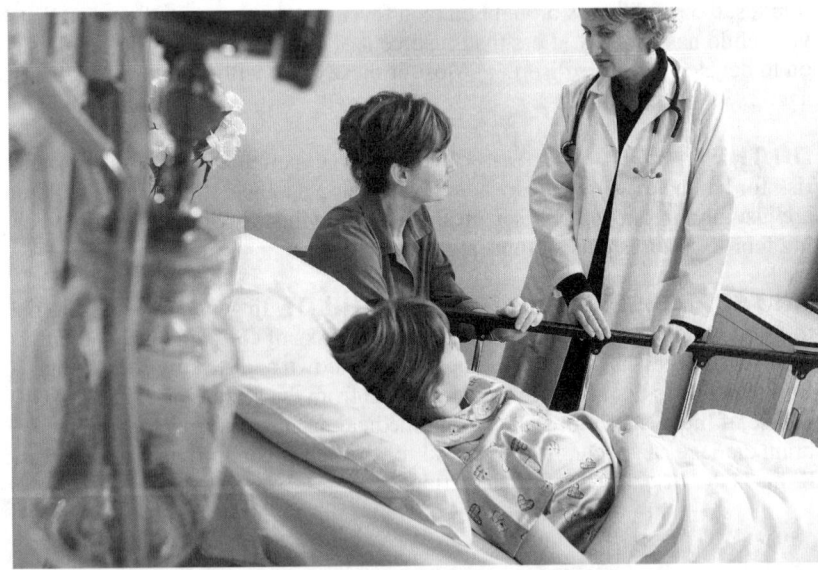

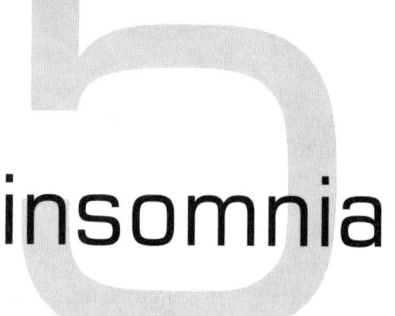

insomnia

HOW MUCH SLEEP IS TOO MUCH AND HOW TIRED IS TOO TIRED? Did you know that 70 million Americans suffer from a sleep disorder and that more than 60 percent of the problems are chronic and long lasting? Did you know that most sleep disorders are distributed evenly among sexes, races, and ages? There are a wide variety of sleep problems, but insomnia is one of the most common.

WHAT IS INSOMNIA? Insomnia is a condition where a person may wake up feeling fatigued and not well rested. This can affect daytime performance and is usually due to insufficient and inadequate sleep.

Symptoms of insomnia include the inability to fall asleep when tired, sleeping very lightly leading to fatigue upon awakening, or waking up too early with the inability to return to sleep.

HOW LONG DOES IT LAST? Insomnia may be temporary, lasting a few days to a few weeks. Transient insomnia will last for a few days, with short-term insomnia lasting for no more than three weeks. Chronic insomnia may last for a very long period of time such as several weeks to months and may include difficulty falling asleep, staying asleep and waking up rested. Usually, there are some primary and secondary identifiable causes of this chronic disorder.

WHAT CAUSES INSOMNIA? The most common cause of transient insomnia is the body's reaction to stress such as dealing with a new illness, injury, death of a loved one or job loss. Other life stressors may also contribute to this problem, but when the stress is removed, the insomnia resolves.

Certain medical conditions such as alterations in hormones during menstruation and pregnancy may contribute to intermittent cases of insomnia. More serious conditions such as cancer, heart disease, thyroid trouble and Alzheimer's disease can contribute to a sleep disorder. Unfortunately, some of the medications used to treat these problems contribute to this as well. These medications can include antidepressants, thyroid medications, seizure medications and beta-blockers.

BRAIN

It is known that nicotine can contribute to sleep disorders. In addition, overuse of alcohol has been proven to disrupt a healthy sleep cycle. Usually a drink or two prior to dinner will not have major impact on the sleep cycle, but may set one up for a restless night.

Lastly, poor sleep hygiene will disrupt the normal circadian rhythm of the body. This is seen most commonly in travelers and shift workers. As an emergency physician, I must adjust to a constant change in my daily routine and with each year of age, it gets a little harder to sleep well after working a night shift. One may not be tired immediately after a night shift and then the sleep cycle may be short and interrupted. This leads to a sense of fatigue later in the day and even the next.

HOW IS THIS TREATED? Initially, the problem must be identified and addressed, leading to the restoration of healthy sleep. There is no one best way to address this problem. Some self-help measures may work. This would include a program of good sleep hygiene.

Some tips that work include establishing a routine for bedtime and sleep, as well as morning awakenings. The bed should not be used as an office. Avoid early evening naps. Exercise is important, but not before bedtime. Avoid eating before bedtime, and this includes alcohol. Avoid large amounts of fluids and caffeine. Do not watch the clock. If you cannot fall asleep within 20 to 30 minutes, get up and read. Usually within a half hour, you may stumble off to bed.

WHAT ELSE CAN BE DONE? With severe and chronic cases, you may need to involve a health care professional. There are physicians that specialize in treating sleep disorders. They will first identify any underlying medical problems that may be contributing to insomnia. This may be done by a sleep questionnaire, medical history and physical examination.

Further testing may involve blood work and a sleep study. The sleep study is conducted in a lab where a patient will spend the night while being monitored. Recommendations may be made on the basis of this study. Sleep aides may be prescribed, but this is done very cautiously, as there are side effects from this treatment.

If you suffer from a sleep disorder, try some of the simple tips that have been outlined. If that does not work, you may need to a see a sleep specialist who may change your life and your nights!

intracranial hemorrhage (ICH)

Israel's former Prime Minister, Ariel Sharon, suffered a transient ischemic attack (TIA). This was a "mini-stroke" and he appeared to have recovered as the symptoms resolved. Then he suffered a major stroke that was hemorrhagic. There are two types of strokes, with the most common being called an ischemic stroke. This is due to a blood clot blocking a blood vessel leading to a lack of blood to the brain.

Sharon suffered a second more serious, and less common, form of stroke that is referred to as hemorrhagic, meaning that actual bleeding is occurring in the brain. This type of stroke accounts for about 12 percent of all strokes and has a high mortality rate.

WHAT HAPPENS WITH BLEEDING IN THE BRAIN? There are several types of conditions that occur with bleeding in the brain. A hemorrhagic stroke, which is also called intracranial hemorrhage, occurs when a blood vessel actually breaks, allowing blood to drain out into the brain tissue. The continued trickle of blood begins to fill the brain tissue and it expands.

The skull allows little room for expansion and eventually there is increased pressure around the brain. Left untreated, the expansion will cause a herniation of the brain where it is pushed out the back of the inside of the skull down into the spinal column. This leads to death in a very short period of time.

WHAT ARE THE SYMPTOMS? The presentation of a hemorrhagic stroke may be gradual or dramatic. There may be a sudden onset of very severe head pain. As the bleeding progresses, the level of consciousness may change. A patient may become confused or appear tired. There may be some outward physical signs such as loss of function of an arm or leg. Once again, these symptoms may be mild or quite severe and noticeable.

With a headache, the pain may be from increased pressure in the brain. This will also lead to nausea and vomiting. A migraine headache may present with similar symptoms of nausea and vomiting, but usually this is a previously diagnosed condition. A new headache with severe nausea and vomiting must be evaluated immediately.

BRAIN

Other factors influencing blood vessel rupture may include drug abuse, infections or vessel malformations. There are a whole host of other unusual blood vessel conditions that may make one susceptible to rupturing a vessel.

WHAT IS THE TREATMENT? This truly is an emergency and requires prompt medical attention. In the emergency department, an evaluation will include blood work. Many patients are on blood thinners such as aspirin, Coumadin, or Plavix. Even though they are life-saving medications, they make it difficult to manage the bleeding. Medicine to reverse the blood thinners may be given.

A CT scan of the brain will be completed to assess if bleeding is present and the amount. Consultation with a neurologist and neurosurgeon will occur.

In the interim, blood pressure will need to be controlled with intravenous medications. If there is an altered level of consciousness and vomiting, a patient will be put under general anesthesia and a tube will be placed in the lungs. This will protect the airway and a ventilator will accomplish breathing.

All of these measures were instituted with Prime Minister Sharon prior to going to the operating room. A wide variety of surgical procedures are available to stop the bleeding and relieve the brain of pressure. Then, a period of watchful waiting occurs to assess the extent of the brain damage.

This is a very serious problem and the chance of surviving one month after an intracranial hemorrhage is a little over 50 percent. Survival chances are improved with prompt evaluation and treatment. Most importantly, as with so many conditions, prevention of the problem is essential and this is why long-standing high blood pressure must be taken seriously and treated.

macular degeneration

Over the Thanksgiving holiday, my wife's 97-year-old great aunt had dinner with us. I have known Isabelle for about 16 years and she is quite a woman. Never married, she lived her whole life in Marshfield, Wisconsin. Also interesting, she never got her driver's license and thus, she walked all over town. That is why she is 97 and quite healthy. Up until the last year, she was working at the local craft shop. Unfortunately, she has lost some of her vision over the past year, and has become a prisoner in her own body. She is unable to read, watch TV, or recognize faces beyond a few feet. Fortunately, she can still see well enough to walk around town.

Treating at the Marshfield Clinic, she was diagnosed with age-related macular degeneration. This is a progressive condition that, as the name states, is related to age.

WHAT IS MACULAR DEGENERATION? This is a chronic eye disease that leads to damage of the macula of the eye. In the back of the eye is the retina, which is where you see things. The macula is in the center of the retina and it is responsible for helping you see fine details of your vision. When this is damaged, it makes it hard to read, recognize faces, or drive. This is called central vision, which is what you see in front of you. Seeing on your sides is called peripheral vision.

Macular degeneration is the leading cause of legal blindness in the United States in people over the age of 55. About 10 million Americans suffer from this disease, with nearly 25 percent over the age of 90.

WHY DOES THIS OCCUR? There are two types of macular degeneration, classified as the wet form and dry form. Wet macular degeneration occurs when there is growth of blood vessels in the center of the retina. They eventually leak, bleed and scar the retina. This leads to the loss of vision through the disruption of the central vision.

Most people suffer from the dry form. Several round yellow and white spots develop around the retina. These spots lead to the breakdown of the retina and macula, leading to loss of the fine central vision. This process is much slower and usually results in minimal vision loss.

As the name states, the most common cause is due to aging. Other medical problems such as tobacco abuse, high blood pressure, high cholesterol, vascular disease and exposure to sunlight place a person at risk. Family history also plays a role in this process.

WHAT ARE THE SYMPTOMS? Most people that are in the early and intermediate stages do not have symptoms. When the disease is severe, the most common symptom is blurred vision. There will be the loss of the ability to perceive fine details at a distance and close up. There may be wavy lines and difficulty in perceiving colors. There may be a blind spot.

WHAT SHOULD I DO? If you are experiencing visual problems, you must be seen by a health care provider. You will be referred to an ophthalmologist, who is a physician that specializes in care of the eye. A comprehensive eye exam will occur and a variety of specialty tests will be administered to evaluate the structure and anatomy of the retina and the macula. Once the diagnosis is made, some treatment recommendations will be given to help with the process, but there is no cure.

Smoking cessation is essential to halt the progression of the disease. Some antioxidants in supplements such as zinc, Vitamin A, C and E may help. Visual aides like magnifying glasses, large print and talking devices will help with activities of daily life.

There are several medications under investigation, but none have been shown to significantly help with the process. Laser treatment early in the disease will stop the progression of the degenerative process, whereby the growing blood vessels are destroyed and new ones do not form.

Macular degeneration is a serious health problem in our country today. If you feel that you are experiencing symptoms of this disease, seek medical attention immediately.

mad cow disease

Right now vegetarians across North American are saying, "We told you so", and shaking their finger at the rest of the meat-loving world. Last week the first case of Mad Cow Disease was discovered in Alberta, Canada, causing thousands of cattle to be killed and even more to be quarantined. Canada's process for the testing of Mad Cow Disease has been extremely lax over the past few years, with reports circulating that cows have gone untested for two years while their meat has been processed and sent throughout North America. Does Mad Cow only affect animals or can humans get it? Are we safe in America? Is the testing in the United States up to par? Should I have chicken salad tonight instead of the porterhouse?

WHAT IS MAD COW DISEASE? Mad Cow Disease or bovine spongiform encephalopathy (BSE) is a fatal brain disorder of cows caused by an unknown agent. The cows that are infected by this actually develop a brain that is sponge-like in appearance. Behavior changes in the animal are noticed and the cow will eventually die.

This illness is similar in nature to Creutzfeldt-Jakob (CJD) disease, which is seen in elderly humans. Chronic Wasting Disease (CWD) in deer is very similar to Mad Cow Disease. All three of these diseases are thought to be caused by either a very small virus particle, mobile bacterium particle or an abnormal protein called a prion.

IS THIS A COMMON PROBLEM? BSE was first diagnosed in the United Kingdom in 1995, with 22 cases in 1996. By 2002, there had been a total of 125 cases reported worldwide but none were present in the United States.

WHAT IS THE PRESENTATION? BSE affects cattle, but unfortunately if a human ingests meats infected with BSE, they will become infected. The incubation period for the cow from the time of exposure to the first signs of the disease may be from two to eight years. Once the cow shows clinical signs of the disease, they will die within six months.

Humans that have consumed the infected meat will show symptoms within one year of consumption. Most of the human cases occurred in the United Kingdom or in people who had traveled there and ate the infected meat.

BRAIN

The average age of the infected patient was 29 and the entire disease process lasted a little over a year. All cases were fatal.

WHAT ARE THE SIGNS? Humans that were infected initially presented with new psychiatric symptoms including depression, apathy, anxiety and psychosis. Some patients were delusional and many of the clinical courses were intermittent. Eventually, the disease progressed and affected intelligence and thought. The final stages involved motor function such as gait, involuntary movements and unresponsiveness.

HOW IS IT DIAGNOSED? Laboratory studies and radiographic imaging was generally of little value for the British physicians. Brain abnormalities were noted on MRI. Testing used to diagnose seizures, such as an electroencephalogram (EEG), revealed nonspecific abnormalities.

WHAT IS THE TREATMENT? As of today, there is no known treatment for Mad Cow Disease. All patients that ate meat infected with Mad Cow Disease eventually died. The prevention of eating this infected meat is essential.

ARE WE AT RISK IN THE U.S.? The U.S. Government has taken a strong position on protecting its citizens from exposure to these infected meats. At present, there is a ban on the import of Canadian beef.

The FDA has stringent policies on the importation of foreign meats or remnants of cattle. As a result of these scientifically-based policies, we have not seen any unfortunate cases of infected cattle or humans in the United States. We can feel reassured that the American population is not at risk for this fatal disease.

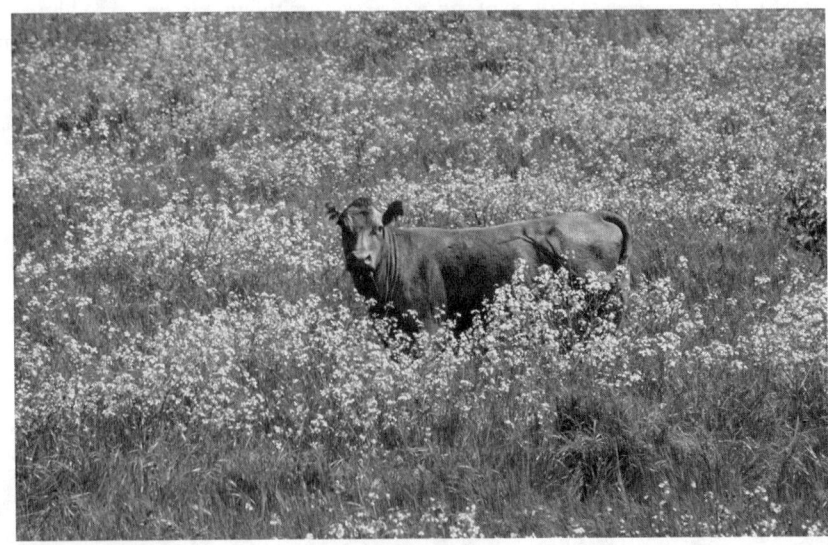

meniere's disease

Have you ever taken a moment to think about just how many diseases are out there? We've covered many well-known or well-documented illnesses in this column, but what about the less familiar or not-yet-documented diseases? Meniere's disease was named after French physician Prosper Meniere in 1861. Well over 600,000 people in the United States have been diagnosed with Meniere's, with 45,000 new cases diagnosed each year.

WHAT IS MENIERE'S DISEASE? This is not an ear infection. Meniere's is a problem with the middle ear and the balance mechanism. There is associated hearing loss as well, in one or both ears. The associated dizziness may be mild to severe.

Dizziness is the sense of light-headedness and unsteadiness. More severe cases involve vertigo, which is a sense that the surroundings are spinning around the person. Meniere's disease is more of a chronic problem, rather than the sudden onset of vertigo, which is usually of much shorter duration.

WHAT ARE THE SYMPTOMS OF MENIERE'S? As noted, Meniere's is a chronic problem that may last for weeks, months or years. A person may experience ear pressure, hearing loss, ringing in the ears, dizziness and vertigo. The onset can be rather abrupt and there may be associated nausea and vomiting. The attacks can last for a long time and a person can have intermittent periods of resolution. The intensities of the attacks can be varied as well. Some people can be symptom-free for months to years.

WHAT ARE THE CAUSES? At the present time, there is no known cause for Meniere's. It is thought that there may be a fluid buildup and pressure in the inner ear. Current research is looking at the effects of chronic noise exposure, viral infections or other biological factors. Researchers are also investigating how the ear perceives sound and converts the energy that is associated with that process.

BRAIN

HOW IS IT DIAGNOSED? Your health care provider will take a comprehensive history with regard to the symptoms, presentation and other associated conditions. A physical examination is essential to rule out other disease processes. In general, there are no specific physical findings. There are no laboratory studies that are indicative of Meniere's disease.

A CT scan or MRI of the brain may eventually be ordered to evaluate the structure of the brain and associated organs. It is important to rule out a tumor, as this can mimic the symptoms of Meniere's. This may be done to rule out other causes of hearing loss.

With associated hearing loss, an audiogram will be completed to assess the magnitude of the problem. In addition, some very specific tests of the balance system may be ordered. This involves some electrical stimulation of the inner ear and the brain stem. These tests will help to confirm the diagnosis.

WHAT IS THE TREATMENT? There are various treatment modalities and success is gauged by trial and error. The most common dizziness medication prescribed is meclizine, a low dose antihistamine that may stabilize the perception of dizziness and calm the associated nausea. If the patient's blood pressure is elevated, this will probably be treated with a diuretic (water pill). There are some physical therapy maneuvers that may help as well.

In rare cases, a surgical procedure may be performed in order to drain fluid from the middle ear. Some ear structures have been removed from the abnormal side in order for the opposite ear structures to compensate. Surgery is usually a last resort and saved for the most severe and complicated cases.

WHAT ELSE CAN I DO? Since we do not fully understand the disease process, there are no preventative measures. If you are affected, it is important that the correct diagnosis is made. Serious medical conditions must be ruled out as well. You may benefit from meclizine and physical therapy. Avoid loud noises and get up slowly. Most importantly, if you feel that you have this condition, you should seek advice from a qualified medical specialist.

migraines

It was interesting to note all of the excitement and exaggeration around Ben
Affleck's visit to the emergency department in Cambridge, Massachusetts, on
Memorial Day for treatment of his migraine headache. Some of the headlines
stated that he was rushed to the hospital for treatment. I don't quite equate the
magnitude of his problem with someone having a heart attack or stroke. But,
migraines are a common problem and about 13 percent of Americans suffer from
these.

Rarely does a shift pass in the emergency department without a migraine headache patient. There are a lot of misconceptions about headaches and migraines,
so let's look a little more closely at issues surrounding the diagnosis and treatment of migraines.

WHAT IS A MIGRAINE HEADACHE? This is a specific type of headache that may be chronic and last for a few hours to a few days. It causes
intense pain, is usually localized to one side of the head and is associated with
other symptoms such as nausea, vomiting, sensitivity to light and noise. Most
importantly, one bad headache does not mean that you suffer from migraines.

There are three different classes of migraines. A migraine with aura used to be
called a classical migraine. This type of headache is associated with an unusual
sensation that precedes the headache. Thus, many people know when they will
get a migraine based on other associated symptoms that occur just prior to their
migraine.

The migraine without aura was called the common migraine. This is the "most
common type" of migraine. This headache comes on with no warning.

The last type of headache is referred to as a migraine variant. These are very interesting, but the symptoms may be frightening. Patients may have visual symptoms, memory problems and even stroke-like symptoms. All of these symptoms
will resolve in a short while and are usually followed by a headache.

BRAIN

WHAT CAUSES A MIGRAINE? There are many theories on the etiology of migraines. It used to be thought that these headaches were caused by a vascular problem, but we have found that this is not the case. It is now thought that migraines are caused by an imbalance of brain chemicals such as dopamine and serotonin.

Stress has been shown to bring on a migraine, as it causes an alteration in brain chemicals. Other factors that may cause a migraine include intense physical activity, travel, lack of sleep, weather changes and a variety of foods. Research has shown that about 100 different foods may lead to the development of a migraine.

WHO GETS MIGRAINES? In the United States, about 30 million people suffer from migraines. Women are affected 3:1 as compared to males. Most migraines peak during the 20-year age group. There is a decline by the time most people reach their 40s. It has been shown that there is a hereditary component as well.

WHAT IS THE TREATMENT? Most importantly, an accurate diagnosis through history and physical examination must be made. A CT scan of the brain will usually be completed to assess brain structure and rule out a tumor. The use of nonsteroidal anti-inflammatory medicines such as ibuprofen works well as initial treatment. Narcotics used to be the mainstay of treatment, but not any longer. Narcotics lead to rebound headaches. Thus, they are dangerous to use and also cause addiction problems.

A wide variety of medications are available to treat a migraine in the emergency department. I start all patients on oxygen. Then, I administer an anti-nauseant medication along with a steroid. My rate of success in alleviating the symptoms is nearly 100 percent. Ultimately, the real treatment involves being able to go home and go to bed.

The approach to migraine treatment was revolutionized about 10 years ago with the advent of the sumatriptan pharmaceuticals. These medications work on brain chemicals and can be easily used at home as a shot, pill, or nasal spray.

Prevention of migraines occurs with use of the high blood pressure medications such as beta-blockers or a calcium channel blockers. These are prescribed in a very low dose and highly effective. If you think that you suffer from migraines, you must be evaluated. There are numerous treatments that can improve your quality of life.

restless leg
syndrome
(RLS)

DO YOU HAVE TROUBLE KEEPING YOUR LEGS STILL? Do you feel like you have ants crawling on your legs? Do you have trouble falling asleep at night? Does your partner complain that you are fidgety when you fall asleep and throughout the night? Have medical tests not revealed any cause for those sensations and medicines not helped? Do other immediate family members have similar symptoms or complaints? You may have Restless Leg Syndrome (RLS) and not even know it.

WHAT IS RESTLESS LEG SYNDROME? RLS is a neurological disorder that is characterized by unusual sensations in the thighs and calves. The sensations may feel like insects crawling on the skin, burning or tugging. The abnormal sensation may be bothersome, irritating and even painful. The best way to alleviate these sensations is to move the legs in a rapid and repetitive fashion. Activity seems to lessen the symptoms and many times the symptoms are worse at night.

HOW COMMON IS RLS? About 8 percent of all Americans suffer from RLS, which equates to about 12 million people. This figure may be low, as this is a fairly common condition that may go undiagnosed and unreported. It is interesting to note that there is a hereditary factor associated with RLS and that 50 percent of all cases have a genetic association among family members.

WHAT IS THE CAUSE OF RLS? Research continues into the causes of RLS and several answers are speculative. There are no known specific causes. As previously noted, there is a hereditary predisposition.

It has been shown that patients with RLS may suffer from anemia and low levels of iron. There may be some underlying medical conditions that contribute to the symptoms such as kidney disease, diabetes, Parkinson's disease and peripheral neuropathy (numbness). During pregnancy, women may experience the symptoms during their last trimester. Lastly, certain cold medications, antiseizure medications, psychiatric medications, some blood pressure medications and antinausea medicines may also worsen the condition.

BRAIN

HOW IS THIS DIAGNOSED? At present, there is no specific diagnostic test that will confirm RLS. A patient must have a comprehensive history taken and physical examination by a health care provider. There are no blood tests that will aid the diagnosis. After all underlying medical conditions have been ruled out the following four basic criteria must be met.

These criteria include: 1) desire to move limbs when there is an associated unusual sensation 2) symptoms that are worse at rest and improved with activity 3) motor restlessness, and 4) symptoms that are worse at night when trying to sleep. The International RLS study group has developed these criterions.

HOW IS THIS TREATED? There is not a standard treatment regimen for RLS. It is important to treat any underlying disease. This would include the use of iron in the treatment of anemia. There may be an electrolyte imbalance of potassium or calcium, and this would need to be addressed. Some high blood pressure medications such as calcium channel blockers may worsen RLS, so they would need to be changed.

A patient may need to work with a doctor that specializes in sleep disorders. A sleep study may be completed and recommendations for sleep hygiene will be made. It is important to develop a regular pattern for sleep, avoid exercise just prior to bedtime, avoid the use of alcohol, be sure to allow for relaxation at bedtime, and avoid complicated mental tasks before bed.

Research has shown that some medications may help. These medicines include those used to treat Parkinson's disease, sedatives, pain relievers and anticonvulsants. None is considered a standard of treatment, but they may help to improve the condition.

WHAT SHOULD I DO? Most importantly, an appropriate diagnosis must be made. Once a diagnosis is made, it is essential to develop a support network. Do not fight the disease, but develop ways to deal with it. Keep a sleep diary and maintain good sleep hygiene. Occupy your mind. Remain active. But most importantly, reach out and help others with a similar problem.

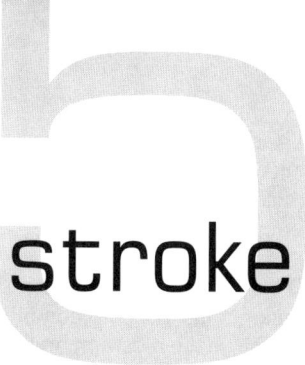

stroke

If you think the only people suffering from strokes are in their senior years, guess again. Every year, over 700,000 Americans suffer a stroke, and range in age from 18 to 100. Strokes are the third leading cause of death and disability in our country, with 20 percent of the victims dying within the first year, at a cost of $30 billion in health care.

WHAT IS A STROKE? A stroke is the reduction of blood flow to the brain. This may be caused by a blood clot blocking an artery supplying the brain with blood. This is called an ischemic stroke. Another type of stroke may be due to the rupture of an artery causing bleeding within the brain. This is called a hemorrhagic stroke.

Both types of stroke cause damage to the architecture of the brain and these brain cells will die when deprived of oxygen-rich blood flow. This process may continue for hours. The ischemic stroke may be more aggressively treated initially, as opposed to the hemorrhagic stroke. It is therefore important to understand the signs and symptoms, so that emergent treatment will be sought.

WHAT ARE THE SIGNS AND SYMPTOMS? It is essential to understand that the signs and symptoms of stroke because they can be very nonspecific and vague. Patients may complain of having a headache or confusion. There may be blurred vision or loss of vision. Additionally, patients may complain of numbness or tingling. There may be difficulty with speech and swallowing. The arms and legs may be numb, weak, or not able to move. Patients may pass out.

It is easy to see that there are numerous signs and symptoms. Most patients will have a few of the above signs. The health care provider must be suspicious of a stroke based on the history of the condition, as well as other risk factors.

WHAT ARE RISKS FOR STROKE? Patients that are at risk for a stroke may have several factors that contribute to the condition. Age is a risk factor and the older the patient, the greater the chance of stroke. Patients who have high blood pressure, are smokers, have diabetes and are overweight have the highest incidence of stroke. The role of high cholesterol in stroke is not clear.

BRAIN

One-and-a-half million Americans suffer from atrial fibrillation, a heart beat rhythm disturbance, and this increases the chance of stroke six-fold! Patients who remain in atrial fibrillation must have their blood thinned through the use of aspirin or warfarin (Coumadin).

WHAT SHOULD I DO? It is essential for patients to modify their risk factors prior to suffering a stroke. This can be accomplished through the help of your health care provider. This is the most important step in dealing with this potentially deadly disease.

In the event that you or a friend experiences the signs of stroke, IMMEDIATE medical attention is necessary. Call 911! The emergency medical technicians will notify the emergency department of the impending arrival of the patient. This will allow the staff to prepare medications and testing.

WHAT SHOULD I EXPECT AT THE HOSPITAL? The diagnosis of stroke must be made in a very timely fashion. A CT scan of the brain will be immediately obtained to determine the nature of the cause. If the stroke is caused by lack of blood supply and not bleeding, a clot-busting drug will be given. This will dissolve the blood clot causing the stroke. This will be done in the emergency department in consultation with the emergency physician and a neurologist. The drug is only effective and safe if given within a three-hour window of the beginning of the symptoms.

Additional medications may also be given to thin the blood. Other studies such as an EKG, blood work, echocardiogram, and carotid dopplers will be obtained during the hospitalization.

HOW LONG IS RECOVERY? As with any medical condition, recovery periods depend on the extent of the damage. Additionally, underlying causes of the medical condition and risk factors must be addressed. A period of physical therapy and rehabilitation may ensue for several months to return the patient to their pre-stroke condition.

Most importantly, it is important for the patient and family to initially recognize the signs and symptoms of stroke. Immediate medical attention will shorten the course of the recovery and decrease the possibility of major disability. It is always imperative to seek medical attention when you are confronted with questions surrounding a stroke.

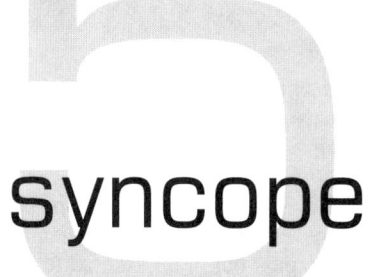

syncope

Before going to church, have something to drink and eat.
If you are feeling faint, sit or lay and put up your feet.

Each Sunday morning, when working in the emergency department, I see a patient that comes in with what I call "Church Syncope." This is a diagnostic phrase that I have coined over the years due to its common occurrence.

What is "Church Syncope?" This is when a person passes out in church during a Sunday service. It happens often and has probably been viewed or experienced by many of our readers. Nationally, about 3 percent of all emergency department visits are the result.

Syncope is a brief loss of consciousness, also referred to as a simple faint. It occurs because the brain is lacking appropriate and adequate blood flow due to a variety of conditions. The body's natural response is to lie down, thereby restoring adequate blood flow to the brain.

Syncope is not only related to the Sunday morning church service, but can present during a variety of activities. It just seems that there is a higher frequency of visits for syncope on Sunday mornings.

WHAT CAUSES SYNCOPE? The causes of syncope are numerous, and many times benign, but must be appropriately investigated. In general, the elderly are more frequently afflicted by syncope and underlying medical conditions can be responsible.

Overall, most syncope is caused by loss of postural tone. This may be secondary to dehydration which may be due to lack of fluid intake or internal bleeding.

Causes of significant concern may be the possibility of a heart arrhythmia, or an unusual heartbeat. The heart may be beating too slow, too fast or irregularly. Many patients may experience a long pause in the heartbeat, which can be very serious. These irregularities alter the amount of blood flow that ultimately reaches the brain.

BRAIN

Other causes of fainting may be related to medications that can slow the heart and lower the blood pressure. Also, neurological issues that affect the brain, such as a stroke, may contribute to this problem.

WHAT SHOULD I DO? The majority of syncope patients have passed out in the past and know when it is going to occur. When they have the premonition that they are going to pass out, it is essential to sit or lie down. It is important to ask for assistance. This will prevent other injuries that can be caused by a fall.

When in a very warm environment, prevent dehydration and drink adequate fluids. Also eat a good breakfast before going to church.

It is very important to realize if you are at risk for syncope. Risk factors include a previous history of fainting, a history of cardiac disease or stroke and taking heart and blood pressure medications that slow the heart rate and lower the blood pressure. Be aware that these risk factors make you a prime candidate for syncope.

WHAT IS THE TREATMENT? As noted before, prevention is essential. It is important that if you feel like you are going to pass out, do not fight that sensation. Ask for immediate assistance to sit or lie down. The feet should be elevated and one should rest quietly until the sensation passes, usually a few minutes.

If someone passes out, be sure that they have not injured themselves in the fall. In addition, be sure that they are lying on a flat surface. It is very helpful to the doctor if the pulse rate is checked. Count the number of beats per minute and determine if the pulse is regular. This is important information when determining the disposition of the patient from the emergency department.

Be sure to call 911 in order to have a timely response of prehospital care providers. Even though it appears that this may be a simple condition, there may be a serious underlying medical cause. The emergency medical technicians are in contact with the doctor at the hospital and can determine if transport is necessary.

WHAT ELSE SHOULD I DO? As always, it is important for your doctor to assess the situation and determine the cause of syncope. Many times, the cause is very simple, but other times it's not. It is important to have an appropriate assessment by you doctor. Remember to take precautions if you know that you are going to be standing for a long period of time, especially if you are taking medications for your heart or blood pressure. Be sure that you eat well prior to going to church and you will not miss the service!

Tinnitus

Over 50 million Americans suffer from tinnitus, yet only 12 million have been diagnosed. Of those diagnosed, about 2 million have difficulty functioning on a day-to-day basis. You may be suffering from this condition and do not even realize what the problem is. Tinnitus is "ringing in the ears" and comes from the Latin derivative of "to tinkle or ring like a bell." This is a not a serious condition, but can be very annoying.

WHAT IS TINNITUS? Tinnitus is the medical term given to someone that perceives an abnormal external or internal sound in the ears. Most commonly, patients complain of a ringing sensation in one or both ears, but patients may experience sounds of chirping, hissing, roaring or clicking.

WHAT CAUSES TINNITUS? There are numerous things that may cause tinnitus and they must all be investigated. This can be a long process involving methodical detective work by your health care provider. There is no known physiological cause, but there are numerous events that can trigger an episode of tinnitus.

Some factors that trigger or worsen the condition include exposure to noise and noise induced hearing loss. Some of the internal ear structures may be damaged by exposure to excessive noise. About 90 percent of people with tinnitus have some sort of associated hearing loss.

Wax buildup and foreign bodies in the ear may contribute to abnormal sounds and sensations in the ears. The buildup can actually lead to a perceived hearing loss, but it can also be an irritant for the disease.

One of the most common causes of tinnitus is aspirin over-dosage. In emergency medicine, physicians are always suspect of aspirin over-dosage. This requires immediate action and treatment. It should be noted that other medications such as Lasix and some antibiotics can cause tinnitus as well.

Some other associated medical conditions such as sinusitis, ear infections, jaw misalignment, heart disease and ear tumors may cause symptoms of tinnitus. All of these potential conditions must be evaluated and ruled out as a source for the disease process.

BRAIN

Many times the treatment involves the removal of the offending factor, such as a medicine, and the condition resolves. Unfortunately, all cases are not easy to diagnose or treat.

HOW IS TINNITUS DIAGNOSED? It is important that the diagnostic process involve a comprehensive history and physical examination. Offending factors need to be clearly identified. Usually, blood tests will be of no value. A hearing test is important, as well as x-ray analysis of the head including a CT scan or MRI. Some cases may require angiography, which is x-ray and dye analysis of the blood vessels of the head and neck. Most importantly, it is essential to remember that the history and clinical course may lead the practitioner to the diagnosis prior to testing.

WHAT IS THE TREATMENT? Fortunately for many individuals, tinnitus will go away on its own in due time. Your health care provider may make some recommendations to speed the recovery period. Initially, if there is an offending factor, such as a medication, it must be stopped. This may lead to complete resolution of symptoms.

For those that are hard of hearing, a comprehensive hearing evaluation is essential. This may lead to the use of hearing aids. Additionally, if there are problems with the jaw and temporomandibular joint, this needs to be addressed.

There are some medications such as antidepressants, antianxiety, antiseizure, and anesthetics that have proven helpful. Your clinician will be able to prescribe one of these medications if appropriate.

A wide variety of other conservative modalities have proven successful. These may include biofeedback and relaxation, use of soft music to combat abnormal sounds and tinnitus retraining therapy (TRT). TRT combines counseling and the use of background sounds. This therapeutic regimen may require 12 to 24 months.

WHAT ELSE SHOULD I DO? If you think that you suffer from tinnitus, you should seek medical attention. For further information, check out the American Tinnitus Association at www.ata.org.

transient global amnesia
(TGA)

An avid reader my column recently experienced a frightening medical event and asked that I write about his condition. Suddenly, without warning, all memory function was lost. Family and friends feared the worst, but within a short period of time, memory functions returned back to normal.

WHAT COULD HAVE HAPPENED TO THIS HEALTHY, MIDDLE-AGED MAN? After a medical evaluation, it was determined that he had suffered from transient global amnesia (TGA). I have seen a few cases of this during my career in the emergency department, so let's look a little more closely at this interesting and fairly benign condition.

WHAT IS TGA? This is a condition where there is a brief and temporary loss of antegrade memory. Antegrade or "forward" amnesia is when a person cannot remember new information. Usually, immediate recall is somewhat preserved, but there is memory loss of recent events and loss of the ability to remember new things. As the name implies, the condition is temporary.

When this occurs, a person may become very frightened and even agitated. They will continue to ask the same question over and over about current happenings. It is interesting to note that there is no loss of ability to speak or use appropriate words. Attention and social skills are retained as well. As the event ends, the affected individual may not recall the events that had occurred during the spell.

WHAT IS THE CAUSE? The exact cause of TGA is not known. It has been recently shown, via a special type of MRI, that blood flow in certain areas of the brain is diminished. This lack of blood supply is only temporary and will not lead to any sort of brain damage. Other associated conditions may mimic TGA. These include: migraine headaches, epileptic seizures and loss of blood flow to the brain as in a mini-stroke (TIA) or stroke. It is known that with a stroke, brain damage will usually occur.

Certain factors may precipitate a TGA attack. These factors include emotional stress, excess physical activity, sexual intercourse, driving and swimming in very cold water.

IS THIS A COMMON CONDITION? Studies completed at the Mayo Clinic have shown that the incidence is about five per 100,000 people in the United States. The rate increases with people over the age of 50, to 23 per 100,000.

WHO IS AFFECTED? Males and females are affected equally and there are no specific race-related factors. As cited, the occurrence increases after the age of 50.

HOW IS TGA DIAGNOSED? Seeking medical attention is essential in order to rule out other more serious problems. The health care provider must take a very detailed and accurate history. The physical examination will usually be fairly unremarkable with the exception of loss of memory function. In the event that there are some remarkable physical findings, TGA may not be the cause of the problem.

Many times, baseline blood tests will be run as well as a CT scan of the brain. It is important to rule out any structural abnormality in the brain such as a tumor or stroke. Usually, a referral to a neurologist is necessary to confirm the diagnosis. An MRI and an EEG (brain wave test) may also be ordered at that time.

WHAT IS THE TREATMENT? Once the diagnosis is made, the patient must be reassured that there is nothing seriously wrong. There are no dietary recommendations or prescription medications that will help in preventing TGA.

To a certain extent, TGA is a diagnosis of exclusion. The health care provider must be vigilant in ruling out any other medical problems. Once this is accomplished, the patient can be reassured that this event will usually not reoccur. In addition, the affected individual is not at risk for developing more serious problems such as a seizure disorder, stroke or brain tumor.

We should be encouraged that ongoing research and the use of advanced radiographic technology may give us better insight into this frightening, but benign condition.

transient ischemic attack (TIA)

The Mayo Clinic published a study which showed that when a patient suffers a Transient Ischemic Attack (TIA) or "mini-stroke," their chances of suffering a stroke with permanent problems within the next three months is 15 percent. This has tremendous implications for both health care providers and patients because a prompt evaluation is essential to improve outcome.

WHAT IS A TIA? This is a temporary lack of blood flow in the brain that can be caused by a variety of factors. The attack is transient and the symptoms will go away within minutes to hours. The symptoms may wax and wane or they may return causing permanent damage. When this occurs, this event is called a stroke.

HOW DOES THIS HAPPEN? The risks of developing a TIA may be due to the narrowing of blood vessels caused by atherosclerosis. The narrowed area has plaque present and the development may be due to high cholesterol. When a blood vessel is narrowed, blood may not be able to freely flow through the vessel.

A TIA may also be caused by the breakage of a plaque and a fragment may travel elsewhere, blocking a blood vessel in the brain. Also, a person may have a blood clot in a part of their body. A piece of the clot may break off and travel to the brain. Both of these processes ultimately cause a lack of blood flow to the brain, leading to symptoms.

WHAT ARE SYMPTOMS OF A TIA? The symptoms are all related to brain function. As you are probably aware, each area of the brain controls certain bodily functions. With a TIA, there may be isolated symptoms or multiple symptoms. Those symptoms may include the loss of speech, the loss of function of an arm or leg, generalized weakness, confusion, headache or abnormal sensation on the skin. Usually, these symptoms may present without warning and then resolve.

HOW IS IT DIAGNOSED? It is essential to seek immediate medical attention in the event that you experience any of the above symptoms. Go to the emergency department of your nearest hospital for evaluation. If that is not practical, see your physician.

BRAIN

Your health care provider will obtain a history of the symptoms and perform a comprehensive physical examination. Next, a set of baseline blood tests will be ordered as well as an electrocardiogram. Once it has been determined that you may have suffered a TIA, additional testing will be ordered.

A CT scan of the brain must be completed to look for evidence of any structural abnormality or bleeding. With a TIA, there will usually be no signs of brain damage or bleeding upon initial evaluation. This test is usually completed during the emergency department visit.

Two other very important tests should be completed within 12 hours of the onset of symptoms. These include a doppler ultrasound study of the carotid arteries in the neck to check for narrowing and an echocardiogram (echo) of the heart. The echo is an ultrasound of the heart that checks for structural abnormalities and for the presence of a blood clot in the heart chambers that can result from a heart arrhythmia such as atrial fibrillation.

WHAT IS THE TREATMENT? Once a timely diagnosis is made, your health care provider may refer you to a neurologist, a physician specializing in brain and nerve problems. If there are no problems, you may be placed on aspirin. Additionally, a medication called Plavix™ may be prescribed to help with blood clotting.

In the event that other structural abnormalities are identified in the blood vessels of the neck, surgery may be necessary. Also, if you suffer from atrial fibrillation, your heart rate will be controlled and you may be placed on another blood thinner called Coumadin (warfarin).

In summary, a TIA is a very serious problem that requires prompt medical attention. A comprehensive workup is essential that will lead to appropriate treatment and hopefully prevent long-term disability.

traumatic
brain injury
(TBI)

Several national and international studies have shown that motorcycle helmets do prevent facial fractures and traumatic brain injuries (TBI). Studies have shown that helmets do not lead to an increase in neck injuries. The psychological, social and financial impact of TBI is staggering.

WHAT IS A TRAUMATIC BRAIN INJURY? This occurs when the brain is subjected to a sudden and violent force, which sends the brain catapulting within the skull, similar to a pinball on a game machine. When this happens, the injury is referred to as closed head trauma.

There may be significant force to break the skull from blunt trauma or from a projectile such as a bullet or rock. These types of injuries are very serious, but less common. The clinical course is much different and the outcome is usually poor. I will not focus on this type of injury in this section.

Each year, about 1.5 million Americans suffer a TBI. About three quarters of these injuries result in mild concussions. But it is important to remember that the brain is sensitive and there may be some long-term problems associated with a brain injury.

WHAT ARE THE SYMPTOMS? As you are aware, the brain controls all thoughts, movements, feelings, sensations and personality. Even the slightest injury can alter these functions. After a blow to the head, there may be some immediate problems.

These symptoms may include a loss of consciousness, confusion, dizziness, memory loss and a headache. There may be other associated injuries, such as a neck injury. Depending on the force, there may be bruising of the brain, bleeding, damage to nerve connections or swelling. The problem associated with swelling is that the brain is contained within a confined space. When this occurs, a patient may experience significant alterations in mental status, severe headache, nausea, vomiting and fatigue. As the swelling progresses, there may be pupil changes, seizures and unconsciousness. This can even lead to death.

BRAIN

WHAT SHOULD I DO? In the event that head trauma occurs, you must seek medical advice immediately. A majority of the cases that we see are minor in nature and only require observation. But an evaluation of the risks, mechanism of injury and physical condition of the individual must be assessed.

Usually, with a significant injury, a CT scan of the brain will be completed to look for structural damage. There may be evidence of bruising of the brain, swelling or bleeding. When this occurs, hospitalization will be required. If the brain is cramped in the skull, surgery may be necessary to relieve the pressure.

WHAT ARE THE LONG-TERM COMPLICATIONS? A wide variety of problems may persist after a TBI. These can include headaches, difficulty concentrating, personality changes and seizures. Several patients will require a fairly long course of rehabilitation in a specialized program for brain-injured individuals. Seizures will need to be controlled with medications. Patients and families may also need to attend counseling to deal with the after effects.

WHAT ELSE CAN I DO? Prevention of a TBI is the most important solution to this problem. The following tips are easy to follow: Always wear a seat belt when driving; be sure that all children are buckled up and in car seats; always wear a helmet when riding a bicycle, skateboard, motorcycle, ATV or snowmobile. Unfortunately, alcohol and drugs play a role in many of these accidents, so avoidance is essential.

Be sure to safety proof your home to avoid falls. The elderly are at an increased risk for TBI as they have less reserve and many are on blood thinners, which lead to bleeding in the brain. A large majority of these injuries are preventable; so take a little extra time to protect yourself.

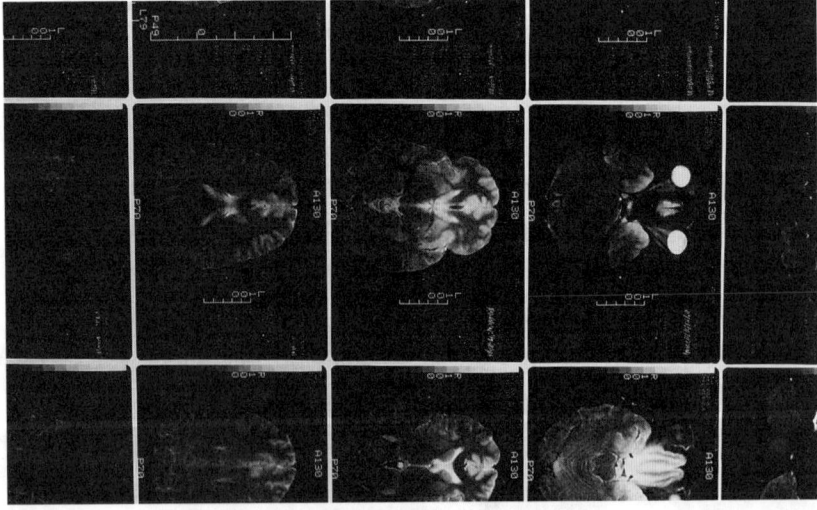

To Your Health with Dr. Wojo

chronic lymphocytic leukemia (CLL)

The reports of news correspondent Ed Bradley touched a lot of people's lives. Even his closest friends and colleagues were shocked at his untimely death due to leukemia. Because of his age, I assumed that he succumbed to chronic lymphocytic leukemia (CLL), a common blood disorder seen in the elderly.

WHAT IS CLL? CLL is a form of cancer that affects bone marrow. Bone marrow is the sponge-like material that is located in the center of the long bones. This is where blood cells are formed. Thus, CLL is a type of blood cancer where there is an abnormally high production of a white blood cell type called a lymphocyte.

The lymphocyte is responsible for fighting off infection when it is functioning normally. But, with this disease process, there are an abnormally high amount of these cells and they gather in the bone marrow, in addition to the liver and spleen. Eventually, they may also gather in the lymph nodes and thus one will see swelling in these areas. When there are really high numbers of lymphocytes, they may interfere with the normal production and function of the red blood cells and the platelets.

WHO GETS CLL? It is interesting to note that this disease is thought to be leukemia of the elderly. More that 90 percent of all patients develop this after the age of 50. In the United States, about 2 people per 100,000 people are affected. There is a higher incidence in Jewish people of Eastern European decent. CLL is virtually nonexistent in Asians.

WHAT ARE THE SIGNS AND SYMPTOMS? Actually, there are no specific signs and symptoms that lead to the diagnosis. Many times, a diagnosis is made on routine physical examination that involves some blood work. The white blood cell count will be high with no other symptoms. But as the disease progresses, other symptoms may become apparent.

CANCER

There may be enlarged lymph nodes, liver and spleen. These organs may be quite obvious on physical examination. A patient may feel weak, fatigued and dizzy. Due to interference with platelet function, there may be a lot of bruising and prolonged bleeding. This may result in anemia, which is a low red blood cell count. At this stage, treatment may be directed at some of the associated problems.

WHAT IS THE TREATMENT? Once the diagnosis is made through the presence of an abnormally high white blood cell count, further staging is necessary to determine the extent of the disease. The Rai System or the Binet System is used to classify the extent of the disease. Many times, there is no treatment needed and patients may survive up to 20 years. The staging system yields a prognosis for survival. Low risk has an average survival of 12 years, intermediate risk 7.5 years and high risk 1.5 years.

Depending on the stage and health of the patient, a variety of modalities may be used. These may include chemotherapy, radiation, steroids, immunotherapy and even bone marrow transplant. All of these treatments may be used individually or in combination. A variety of factors come into play when making this decision. Many times, no treatment is necessary as the disease process is less harmful than the treatments available.

Usually, a patient that is younger will require an aggressive form of treatment. Recent studies have shown that bone marrow transplant has been quite effective in eradicating the disease.

WHAT ELSE CAN BE DONE? If you are diagnosed with CLL, you will need to explore your options with your health care provider. You may be referred to a cancer specialist for additional evaluation. Keep yourself healthy and be sure to get immunizations like the flu shot. Patients with CLL are at increased risk for developing infections. You may need to seek medical attention much sooner than normal for treatment of a fever, sore throat or respiratory illnesses. Exercise and maintain a healthy diet.

There is continued research into different protocols and patients can enroll in the latest treatment regimens. Additional information can be found at www. inh.gov.

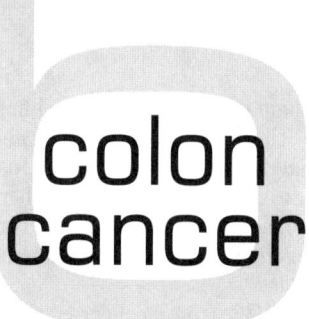

colon cancer

March is National Colon Cancer Awareness month and celebrities promote preventative medicine through public appearances, including televised colonoscopy. Katie Couric's husband died from colon cancer and Sharon Osbourne is a survivor.

WHAT IS COLON CANCER? Cancer of the colon can occur in any part of the large intestine or the rectum. An uncontrolled growth of cancerous cells will invade the walls of the colon leading to a disruption of blood flow inside the intestine. The colon consists of four to five feet of the large intestine, with the last four to five inches being the rectum.

Colon cancer is the fourth leading cancer in both men and women. In men, the most common cancers are skin, prostate, lung and colon. In women, the most common cancers are skin, lung, breast and colon. In both sexes, colon cancer usually occurs after the age of 50 years.

HOW DOES IT OCCUR? The causes of colon cancer are not completely known, but there are some known risk factors. These factors include increased age, history of colon polyps, family history of colon cancer, some genetic conditions, diet and smoking.

Cells within the lining of the intestine continue to develop, grow and eventually die off. When some of those cells do not die off, they continue to grow and develop a tumor. Many of these cells have an abnormal makeup, which are cancer cells. The cancer cells continue to replicate leading to a large growth. Colon polyps are growths of tissue within the lining of the intestine. They can be benign or cancerous. These growths must be removed and checked for cancer. Many colon cancers arise from colon polyps.

WHAT ARE THE SYMPTOMS? A person with early colon cancer may have no symptoms and the cancer may be found incidentally on physical examination where a trace amount of blood is seen in the stool sample. When this occurs, the health care provider will pursue a search for colon cancer. Blood in the stool may indicate a possibility of cancer, but there are many causes for blood in the stool such as ulcers or hemorrhoids.

CANCER

Some patients may complain of a change in bowel habits such as increased constipation or diarrhea. There may be bloating or abdominal pain. Later stages of colon cancer may lead to weight loss and loss of appetite. In addition, blood work may show evidence of anemia. There are no very specific symptoms of colon cancer, so a health care provider must put all the pieces of the big clinical picture together in order to make the diagnosis.

HOW IS IT DIAGNOSED? Colon cancer is diagnosed on the basis of the history and physical examination. Hereditary factors must be considered as well. Screening for colon cancer usually starts with checking the stool for small amounts of blood that cannot be seen by the naked eye.

Additional screening may lead to a flexible sigmoidoscopy or colonoscopy. A doctor will use a flexible lighted scope to inspect the inside of the colon. This can be done in the doctor's office or the hospital. Sedation will be given in order make the procedure more comfortable.

There are some x-ray tests that may be ordered, such as a barium enema, in order to identify any abnormalities. A CT scan of the abdomen may be ordered to check for the spread of cancer. Lastly, some blood work may be obtained to check for abnormalities in blood chemistries, but there are no diagnostic blood tests to screen for colon cancer.

WHAT IS THE TREATMENT? Depending on the extent of the colon cancer, a variety of treatments are available including surgery to remove the cancerous growth. Additional chemotherapy and radiation may be necessary. This all depends on the size and extent of the cancer.

Several medical specialists may be consulted in order to provide the most current and effective treatment based on the specific case. You may wish to seek a second opinion as well, and your primary care provider will help facilitate in order to provide the best care possible. Remember, early diagnosis leads to full recovery in many cases. Be sure to seek preventative medical care, as this may save your life!

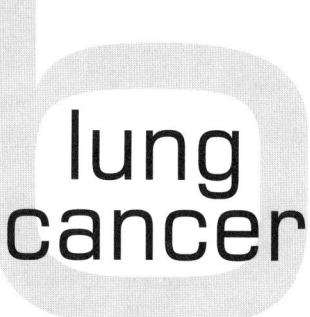

lung cancer

Peter Jennings, 67, died from lung cancer that was diagnosed in April 2005 and was caused by a lifetime of smoking. Shortly after his death, the widow of Christopher Reeve, Dana Reeve, announced that she had lung cancer. Reeve, a nonsmoker– which is unusual– died despite aggressive treatment less than a year after the diagnosis.

WHAT IS LUNG CANCER? Lung cancer is a malignant tumor of the lungs that is divided into two primary types called non-small cell and small cell carcinoma. About 80 percent of all lung cancer is the non-small cell type, which is not as aggressive and grows more slowly. There are numerous subtypes of non-small cell cancer, determined on the basis of the actual cell type that is identified after a biopsy.

Small-cell carcinoma is a little more rare, but very aggressive. It has also been called oat cell carcinoma. This cancer has a greater chance of spreading to other parts of the body's organs. Thus, a rating called staging, will address if the cancer has stayed in the chest or spread to other body areas. The smaller the stage number, the greater the chance of survival.

HOW COMMON IS LUNG CANCER? In the United States, it is projected that there will be about 173,000 new cases of lung cancer each year. Unfortunately, about 94 percent, or 163,000, patients will die. The demographics have improved for white and black men, but worsened for white and black females. Since 1987, the death rate of lung cancer has surpassed the death rate of breast cancer in women. Overall, lung cancer is still the leading cause of cancer deaths in both sexes.

WHAT CAUSES LUNG CANCER? As soon as I heard of the diagnosis of lung cancer in Jennings and Reeve, I assumed that both were smokers. Unfortunately, for Reeves, she was in a very small minority of non-smokers that develop lung cancer.

The leading cause of lung cancer is smoking and about 90 percent of all cases are seen in smokers. Tobacco is filled with cancer-causing agents that will damage the lungs, leading to the development of cancer. The longer and the more frequently a person smokes, the greater the chance will be that they develop lung cancer. This is even true of cigar and pipe smokers.

Continued studies address the issue of second-hand smoke and lung cancer. It has been shown that this is a risk factor as well. This is also referred to as involuntary or passive smoking.

Chemical exposures increase one's risk for developing lung cancer. These chemicals may include radon gas or asbestos. Radon gas comes from the soil and rocks, and may be found in some homes. Asbestos is a fiber that was used in older insulation, manufacturing, brake repair and shipbuilding. The particles of asbestos break down and float into the lungs, thus leading to the development of a tumor.

WHAT ARE THE SYMPTOMS? Usually, a health care provider will be suspicious of lung cancer in a patient who is a smoker or has other risk factors. Possible symptoms of lung cancer may include a chronic cough, increasing shortness of breath, wheezing, chest pain, loss of appetite or unexplained weight loss. Other signs of lung cancer may be weakness, bloody and productive cough, unusual bone pain, hoarseness or difficulty swallowing.

HOW IS IT DIAGNOSED AND TREATED? Clinical suspicions by a health care provider will usually lead to blood work and a chest x-ray. If an abnormality is seen on a chest x-ray, a CT scan is usually ordered. Once a mass or tumor is seen, a bronchoscopy may be performed to gather some tissue. Bronchoscopy involves looking into the lungs with a fiber optic tube.

When the diagnosis is made, surgery may be done to remove the tumor. Also, a combination of radiation and chemotherapy may be prescribed. Several different regimens are available depending on the specific diagnosis of the patient. Therapy is quite intensive.

Prevention is essential; as lung cancer is so deadly, quit smoking immediately! This will improve your chances of not developing lung cancer and having a full life span!

male breast cancer

On July 1, 2004, a national study was released that alerted us to the prevalence of male breast cancer in the United States. Once thought of as a nonexistent disease, the study will confirm that men do get breast cancer. About 1,600 men each year in the United States are diagnosed with this serious disease. The study showed that the incidence of male breast cancer has risen about 25 percent in the past 25 years. It has been thought that about 0.25 percent of all men will be affected.

WHAT IS MALE BREAST CANCER? Male breast cancer is a malignant tumor of the tissue in the cells of the breast. Men have ducts in the breast just like women but the tissue is not as pronounced due to the male hormones that control their growth. This tissue or the nipple can become cancerous.

IS THIS SIMILAR TO FEMALE BREAST CANCER? Yes. There are many similarities between male and female breast cancers. Women are at least one hundred times more affected than males. Also, at present, there is much greater awareness and sensitivity for female breast cancer. Due to the growing incidence of male breast cancer, health care providers are addressing this issue with males.

As for women, adenocarcinoma is the most common form of breast cancer. There are many different descriptions used based on location and extent of the cancer. For example, carcinoma-in-situ is more localized in the breast as opposed to infiltrating or invasive carcinoma.

WHAT ARE THE RISKS FOR MALE BREAST CANCER? It is not clear what actually causes male breast cancer. It is known what associated risk factors will predispose a man to developing breast cancer.

The aging process increases the risk for male breast cancer. The average age of a man with the diagnosis is 68 years, as opposed to 63 years for a woman. Male breast cancer has been diagnosed from ages 5 to 93 years.

The second most common risk factor is genetics. A positive family history of male and female breast cancer significantly increases one's risk for this disease process. There are a variety of genes that can mutate and lead to the development of the cancer.

Some other known risk factors that are associated with the development of male breast cancer include exposure to radiation. This may be related to radiation treatment for other cancers. Men with liver disease have an alteration in proteins that carry sex hormones. It is known that alterations in sex hormones such as testosterone can be associated with the development of this cancer. Also, hormonal treatment with estrogen may increase the risk as well.

HOW IS IT DIAGNOSED? Male and female breast cancers follow the same diagnostic process. A comprehensive history and physical examination are essential. The presence of a lump, a draining sore or a change in the nipple may be an indication of an underlying cancer. Early diagnosis leads to a better outcome whereby the five-year survival rate is 98 to 99 percent in these cases. Diagnostic testing may include some laboratory studies and x-rays. A mammogram or ultrasound of the tumor will help localize the problem.

Once this is done, a needle biopsy or surgical biopsy will confirm the diagnosis. A pathologist, who will make the final specimen diagnosis, will evaluate the tissue in the lab.

WHAT IS THE TREATMENT? Treatment may include surgical removal of the tumor or the breast. Lymph nodes will be assessed and chemotherapy may be recommended. Additionally, radiation may be another modality used to treat the cancer. Depending on the type of tumor, long-term hormonal therapy may be indicated as well.

An oncologist, a physician specializing in the treatment of cancer, will determine all of these treatment protocols. There are numerous regimens that can be used based on the type of cancer.

WHAT ELSE SHOULD I DO? Contrary to popular thought, males do develop breast cancer. In the event that a lump is felt on or around the breast, it must be thoroughly investigated. This is a very serious disease, but if caught early, the chances of survival are great.

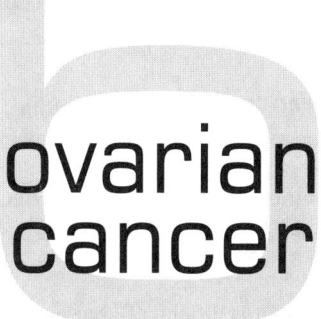

ovarian cancer

Each September, medical professionals attempt to enhance the awareness for ovarian cancer in females. Ovarian cancer is very serious with a grim outlook, but the statistics for American women are improving. This is a difficult cancer to diagnose, but health care providers must be cognizant of the potential for diagnosis.

WHAT ARE THE OVARIES? The two ovaries are small almond-shaped organs that are located next to the uterus and just above the bladder. They are the center of the reproductive system of women. Each ovary stores between 200,000 and 400,000 follicles that help form an egg.

During the reproductive cycle, a follicle within the ovary will rupture and release an egg. The egg moves down the fallopian tube into the uterus, where the male sperm may fertilize it. If this does not happen, the egg is discarded as a product of the menstrual cycle.

Ovaries are also responsible for the secretion of estrogen and progesterone. These hormones may be medically replaced when the ovaries are removed. Hormonal replacement has been identified as a possible risk factor for the development of ovarian cancer.

WHAT IS OVARIAN CANCER? Ovarian cancer is the development of a neoplasm or tumor on one or both of the ovaries. The exact cause of this cancer is unknown, but risk factors have been identified.

Each year, over 23,000 American women are diagnosed with ovarian cancer and over 50 percent die from this fairly uncommon cancer. It is the fifth leading cause of cancer death in women and the leading cause of death from gynecologic cancers.

There are three types of tumors that develop and the most common is an epithelial tumor. The other two less frequent types of tumors are called germ cell and stromal. Each tumor develops in a different part of the ovary, thereby categorizing it by name.

WHAT ARE THE SYMPTOMS? The symptoms of ovarian cancer are very, very nonspecific and unfortunately in many cases, by the time the diagnosis is made, the cancer has spread. Patients may complain of abdominal discomfort, nausea, abdominal fullness, pelvic heaviness, constipation, loss of appetite, unexplained weigh loss or gain and possibly abnormal vaginal bleeding.

The average age of the patient is around 60, but ovarian cancer can afflict women ages 20 to 90. The risk of any female getting ovarian cancer with no risk factors is a little over 1 percent.

HOW IS IT DIAGNOSED? As noted, ovarian cancer is very difficult to diagnose because of the nonspecific symptoms. Health care providers must be suspicious when evaluating at-risk females. The history and physical examination are the initial diagnostic tools. The physical examination includes a pelvic examination and bimanual exam, where the clinician actually feels the ovaries. Further testing will include ultrasound and blood testing for tumor markers. If the disease has spread, a CT scan will be necessary to quantify the spread of the cancer. Unfortunately, the diagnosis is many times made after the extensive spread of the cancer.

WHAT ARE RISK FACTORS? Women at risk include those with a positive family history of ovarian cancer. Other factors include the presence of a previous cancer such as breast cancer, having never been pregnant, smoking, hormone replacement and diet.

WHAT IS THE TREATMENT? Initially, your gynecologic surgeon will make the diagnosis and determine the spread of the disease. Once this is accomplished, staging of the disease will determine how extensive the cancer is and where it is located. Most treatment includes the removal of the cancerous ovaries and possibly other cancerous organs.

After surgical removal, which is usually a hysterectomy, chemotherapy is initiated. There are numerous agents that are used and your oncologist will determine which is best on the basis of the type of tumor and staging of the disease. Radiation has not been an option due to the extensive area that would need to be radiated.

prostate cancer

Each September, health care providers focus on a leading cause of cancer in males, which is prostate cancer. Only lung cancer occurs more frequently in males and has a much higher mortality. The risk of a male developing prostate cancer is nearly one in ten. There are less than 200,000 cases diagnosed annually and over 30,000 American males die each year. Prostate cancer is highly curable, but it must be diagnosed early.

WHAT IS THE PROSTATE? The prostate is a male gland that is located between the bladder and rectum. The function is to provide fluid to form semen. It is a smooth and soft muscular gland that surrounds the urethra, which carries urine. It allows for the passage of semen by contracting and not allowing for the passage of urine during sexual intercourse.

WHAT IS PROSTATE CANCER? Prostate cancer is the development of a malignant tumor within the prostate gland. It is very common and over 90 percent of all cases are minor and even go undetected. The risk of the development begins after age 40, but it is more common with aging. By the age of 80, nearly three quarters of all men have prostate cancer.

Fortunately, most cases of prostate cancer are very small and discovery is incidental. A large number of these cases do not require treatment, only careful observation by the health care provider.

HOW IS IT DIAGNOSED? Prostate cancer may initially be diagnosed due to urinary symptoms such as difficulty with urination, blood in the urine, difficulty starting or stopping stream, or back pain. All of these symptoms may be seen with other diseases and not related to prostate cancer.

Physical examination will include a digital rectal exam that may detect the presence of a lump on the prostate. Prior to this exam, a blood test may be completed revealing the evidence of an elevated Prostatic Specific Antigen (PSA). There are a couple of different types of PSA and your hospital's laboratory will choose the most appropriate test.

Prostate cancer releases a very small amount of PSA into the blood that can be detected. Normal reference lab values will be provided in order to help you understand the test. Other tests may include an ultrasound and a biopsy to confirm the diagnosis.

CANCER

WHAT IS THE TREATMENT? Once the diagnosis is made, several options will be presented including "watchful waiting," drug therapy, radiation and surgery. It is important to discuss all of these issues with your doctor. Treatment will depend on the stage of the disease.

Several different classifications have been developed. Most simply, Stage I is very minor and not detected on digital rectal exam. Most of these cases are found incidentally on health screenings including a laboratory study. Stage II involves more tissue of the prostate and can be felt on digital exam. Stage III has spread to tissues surrounding the prostate and Stage IV has spread through the blood stream into other body parts such as the lymph nodes. This last stage is very serious and may require aggressive treatment.

WHAT ARE THE RISK FACTORS? The exact cause of prostate cancer remains unknown. Factors that increase the development of prostate cancer include advanced age, family history, chemical exposure, obesity, smoking, alcohol, lack of exercise and diet. None of the above risk factors have a direct correlation with the development of prostate cancer, but family history is probably most important.

WHAT SHOULD I DO? It is well known that if prostate cancer is detected early, the success of treatment is 98 percent. A digital rectal exam and a lab test are recommended annually after the age of 50.

Incidental discoveries of elevated PSAs can alert your doctor to the need for close observation or more aggressive treatment. The treatment outlines will be presented once a diagnosis is made.

WHAT ELSE CAN I DO? Be sure to practice a healthy life style and limit your risk factors. You cannot choose your family history, but exercising and avoiding smoking and excessive alcohol may improve your chances of not developing the disease. It is important to be evaluated if you develop any urinary symptoms because early treatment is the most successful!

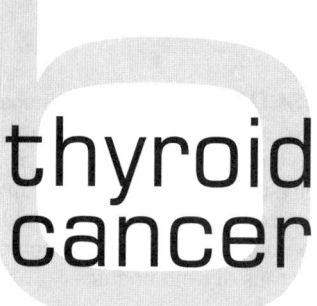

thyroid cancer

The diagnosis and treatment of Chief Justice Rehnquist's thyroid cancer has heightened our awareness of this fairly rare disease. Each year, about 20,000 Americans are diagnosed with thyroid cancer, which accounts for only 5 percent of all thyroid nodules or lumps. Several more people undergo evaluation of thyroid nodules or lumps, and fortunately only a small percentage are cancerous. When diagnosed early, the chances of survival are greater than 90 percent, depending on the type of cancer present.

WHAT IS THYROID CANCER? The thyroid is an endocrine gland that is located in the neck over the Adam's Apple. The gland has a right and left lobe. The function of the gland is to produce thyroid hormone that helps regulate many bodily functions.

The gland may develop nodules. There may be a single nodule or several nodules. When the gland has several nodules, it is referred to as a multinodular goiter. About 95 percent of all nodules are not cancerous, but they require medical evaluation.

When cancer is diagnosed in the thyroid, it may be found in several different forms. The forms are identified by the type of cell in the thyroid in which the cancer arises. The thyroid may have papillary carcinoma, follicular carcinoma, anaplastic carcinoma, medullary carcinoma and thyroid lymphoma. Each type of cancer has its own unique features.

Justice Rehnquist was diagnosed with anaplastic carcinoma, which is an uncommon type. This is usually a very aggressive form of thyroid cancer that can spread in the neck and to other parts of the body. The outlook for survival is not positive when there is spread of this cancer.

WHAT ARE THE SIGNS OF THYROID CANCER? Early signs and symptoms of thyroid cancer are minimal. As the cancer begins to grow, you or your health care provider may feel a lump in the thyroid gland. As the lump begins to grow, there may be pain in the neck that radiates into the throat. There may be a sore throat or some difficulty breathing. Additionally, you may experience unexplained hoarseness or the presence of noticeable lymph nodes in the neck. Usually, there are no other significant signs and symptoms associated with the disease.

HOW IS IT DIAGNOSED? There must be clinical suspicion of thyroid disease and the presence of a nodule will require further evaluation. Blood tests may be performed to check the level of the thyroid hormone. These would be ordered after physical examination of the thyroid gland and a nodule is discovered. A nuclear medicine thyroid scan would then be completed to confirm the presence of a nodule. The thyroid scan does not tell the difference between benign and cancerous thyroid nodules.

Once the nodule is confirmed, a fine needle aspiration (FNA) procedure is performed. A very small needle is used to obtain tissue samples of the thyroid. A pathologist evaluates the samples obtained in order to make the diagnosis. If a diagnosis cannot be made, a surgical biopsy must be taken to confirm the diagnosis.

WHAT IS THE TREATMENT? Usually, benign nodules will require no treatment. If cancer is found, the type must be identified. Usually, thyroid cancer requires removal of the gland by a surgeon experienced in removing it. After that, radiation therapy and/or chemotherapy may be prescribed in order to completely address the problem. The oncologist will outline all of the treatments available for the particular type of cancer present. Ongoing research and protocols will direct this decision.

CAN I PREVENT THE DEVELOPMENT OF THYROID CANCER?
As with most cancers, a healthy life style is encouraged. With a family history of thyroid cancer, preventative removal of the thyroid may be considered. Most importantly, early diagnosis and treatment yields a better outcome, so seek medical attention in the event that you have unexplained neck symptoms or discover a mass in your neck.

aortic aneurysm
(AAA)

As memorial services were held for the victims of 9/11, actor John Ritter lay on an operating table in California, struggling for his life. He succumbed to a ruptured aortic aneurysm, just as so many people do in the United States. If undetected and allowed to rupture, over 80 percent of all people will die.

WHAT IS AN ANEURYSM? The term aneurysm comes from the Greek term aneurysma, which means widening. The widening occurs in a blood vessel, such as the aorta, the largest artery in the body. There is a bulge in a section of the blood vessel, like a worn spot in an old inner tube of a tire. The weakened bulge, which is under pressure from the pumping of the heart, will actually burst causing hemorrhage and death.

HOW DOES THIS OCCUR? The causes of aneurysms are numerous and may include a hereditary component. Hereditary conditions affecting the elasticity of the blood vessels may also be a cause. Patients that have arteriosclerosis, or "hardening of the arteries," are at greatest risk. Additionally, many of these folks have high blood pressure, which is also another major risk factor.

Other causes of aneurysms include a vessel that has been weakened by infection or an inflammatory process. Anyone who has experienced trauma to a great vessel is also placed at tremendous risk for development of an aneurysm.

WHO IS AT RISK? In general, males outnumber females by 5:1 in developing aneurysms. Age is another risk factor and most patients are over the age of 60. If a patient has some of the risk factors listed above, the incidence of aneurismal development is quite high.

WHAT ARE THE SYMPTOMS? Some of the most common symptoms include chest and abdominal pain that will radiate into the back. The pain can have a sudden onset in nature and it may be very severe. In extreme cases, the blood pressure may be low, which indicates that the aneurysm has ruptured and death is eminent.

CARDIORESPIRATORY

HOW IS IT DIAGNOSED? Initially, the health care provider must consider the history and risk factors. Aortic aneurysm should always be a consideration in older patients that present with chest and abdominal pain that radiates to the back. The evaluation includes assessment of vital signs, laboratory studies and ultrasound. A CT scan may also be used in helping make the diagnosis. MRI is not necessary for diagnosis.

HOW IS IT TREATED? The initial incidental diagnosis of an aortic aneurysm involves close monitoring and measurement through ultrasound or CT scan. Aneurysms that are 5 centimeters (about 2 inches) or less are followed by radiographic testing every few months.

When the aneurysm continues to get larger, surgical correction is necessary. Risk for dissection of the aneurysm grows with increased size. The weakened walls of the blood vessel will allow blood to seep in between layers of the blood vessel, which can cause narrowing of the inner size of the vessel. This dissection can lead to rupture and premature death.

Once diagnosed, surgeons will remove the weakened portion of the vessel and replace it with Dacron (plastic-like) tubing, where the damaged vessel previously existed. Recently, the use of stents has been used to help bypass the damaged vessel. Elective surgical correction is quite successful, but emergency surgical correction has a high mortality.

WHAT SHOULD I DO? In the event that you have risk factors for an aneurysm and symptoms, your health care provider must evaluate you. The provider will determine the course of action and order the appropriate tests. Once a diagnosis is made, watchful waiting may ensue. In the event that the aneurysm is large, your health care provider will arrange a visit with a surgeon.

As always, prevention is essential. A healthy lifestyle will promote healthy blood vessels. But, in the event that you have risk factors and symptoms, a visit to your doctor is essential, as it may save your life!

asthma

During spring, a lot of people are bothered by asthma. A friend of mine at the hospital mentioned this to me and asked that I write about this issue. When he said he was having trouble with his asthma, I started to notice that I was seeing a lot more patients that required some management of this respiratory condition.

WHAT IS ASTHMA? This is a chronic respiratory condition that affects the airways of the lungs. The smaller breathing passages, such as bronchioles, become inflamed and irritated. When this happens, these tiny tubes do not allow for appropriate passage of air within the lungs. This results in wheezing that may only be heard with a stethoscope, but more severe cases can actually be audible when you are near a patient.

There are four levels of severity, which are defined by frequency of attacks. Mild Intermittent asthma occurs twice a week or at least two attacks at night during a month. Mild persistent asthma occurs more than twice a week and is brought on by physical activity.

More severe cases are referred to as Moderate Persistent asthma, which occurs daily and at least one night per week. This condition clearly affects physical activity. Lastly, Severe Persistent asthma occurs throughout every day and night with significant limitation in activity.

WHO HAS ASTHMA? In the United States, there are about 17 million people afflicted, with 5 million of these being children. In the 1970s, there was a decline in the condition, but that trend has unfortunately changed.

About 6 percent of African Americans have the disease, as opposed to 5 percent of Americans with European decent. It should be noted that about 5,000 Americans die each year because of asthma, and the death rate among children is fairly high.

WHAT CAUSES ASTHMA? The exact cause of asthma is not clear. The inflammation of the airways can be caused by a variety of factors, but we know that there is also a hereditary link among families.

CARDIORESPIRATORY

Some things that trigger an asthmatic attack include exposure to allergens, infections such as viral illnesses and pollutants like smoke. There is a significant allergic component to the disease, so exposure to animals, dust, pollen and certain odors may trigger an attack. Thus, we see a greater number of emergency department visits during the spring as plants begin to bloom.

WHAT ARE THE SYMPTOMS? Most obvious is wheezing, but a persistent cough, especially at night, may be a clue to the problem. Other patients may have significant trouble breathing with chest tightness. The most severe cases may present with a patient in acute respiratory distress appearing ashen or bluish in color.

HOW IS THIS TREATED? It is important that an appropriate diagnosis is made with an evaluation of the respiratory history. After an acute attack, diagnostic testing may include allergy testing, respiratory function testing, x-rays and even checking for gastroesophageal reflux or heartburn that may irritate the airways.

In the emergency department, a nebulizer or aerosol of a bronchodilator, such as albuterol, may be used. A combination of other medications may be given in nebulizer form. For a majority of the cases, this usually takes care of the problem. More severe cases may require the use of anti-inflammatory steroids given intravenously or taken in pill form.

A patient may be sent home with an inhaler and taught how to use it by a respiratory therapist. The health care provider may order a home nebulizer as well. Lastly, inhaled anti-inflammatory steroids may be ordered in addition to the above treatment. This has become a very important part of outpatient treatment.

Asthma is a common problem, but it can be very serious. Smoking and asthma are a death sentence! If you smoke, you must stop. Most importantly, if you feel that you have asthma, you should be evaluated. Most treatments are very safe and will improve the quality of your lifestyle.

atrial fibrillation

Millions of Americans live with heart ailments on a daily basis. Gone untreated, these disorders may become very serious. One of the more common heart conditions facing Americans today is atrial fibrillation and it is no exception to the rule. When properly treated, people living with this irregular heart rhythm can perform daily activities on a regular basis.

WHAT IS ATRIAL FIBRILLATION? Atrial fibrillation is an irregular heart rhythm disturbance whereby the upper chambers of the heart, the atria, beat in a rather uncontrolled and uncoordinated fashion. In the United States, over 2 million Americans suffer from this disturbance and nearly 5 percent of patients over the age of 69 are affected.

HOW DOES IT OCCUR? The normal electrical impulses that control the heart start in the upper chamber of the right side called the right atrium. This impulse then travels down the center of the heart to the lower chambers, known as the ventricles, causing an even, coordinated pumping action of the upper and lower chambers of the heart.

With atrial fibrillation, the electrical impulse is somewhat distorted and the regular pumping of the atria does not occur. This causes a form of quivering in the upper chambers, which are not synchronized with the lower chambers, affecting the heart's ability to pump blood and causing an increase in heart rate.

WHAT CAUSES ATRIAL FIBRILLATION? Atrial fibrillation can be caused by a number of things. In the younger population, the use of drugs or excessive use of alcohol may be a significant cause.

With an older patient, underlying coronary artery disease secondary to high blood pressure, high cholesterol or diabetes may damage the architecture of the heart. Additionally, the presence of heart valve disease may cause the rhythm disturbance.

Patients that have an overactive thyroid or a lung disease such as emphysema or pneumonia are also at risk. Certain stimulant medications may also cause a change in the heart rhythm. Although these are all underlying causes for atrial fibrillation, some people with no previous risk factors develop the heart rate disturbance.

CARDIORESPIRATORY

WHAT ARE THE SYMPTOMS? The most common symptom of atrial fibrillation is an irregular pulse. A very rapid, irregular pulse may be accompanied by shortness of breath, chest pain, generalized weakness and fatigue. Some patients also complain of light-headedness and feeling faint, while others may be completely asymptomatic and not realize that they have an irregular pulse. Many patients comment that it feels like their pulse is racing and slowing down, palpitating or skipping beats.

HOW IS IT DIAGNOSED? Once a patient develops clinical symptoms, their health care provider will order an EKG, which is a paper heart tracing of the electrical impulses of the heart. Atrial fibrillation has a very specific appearance on an EKG and is quite easily diagnosed. Once this is accomplished, blood tests may be ordered to check for an electrolyte imbalance, overactive thyroid or heart damage. If problems or symptoms continue, your health care provider may order an echocardiogram, which is an ultrasound (sound wave) picture of the heart.

HOW IS IT TREATED? The goal of treatment is to return the heart to its normal rhythm. This can be accomplished through the use of intravenous medications, oral medications or electrical shocking (cardioversion). Many patients will need to be on medication to maintain the normal heart rhythm following treatment.

If a patient remains in atrial fibrillation, they are at increased risk for developing a stroke. To help prevent this from occurring, the health provider may need to thin the patient's blood using Coumadin.

WHAT SHOULD BE DONE? There is not a lot that someone can do to prevent the development of atrial fibrillation, with the exception of limiting risk factors. In the event that you develop an irregular pulse, it is essential you visit your health care provider for an evaluation. The appropriate diagnosis must be made and treatment will be rendered. This can be a fairly benign disease, but left untreated, the consequences can be devastating!

automated external defibrillator (AED)

Each year, about 250,000 Americans die before reaching the hospital after suffering sudden cardiac arrest (SCA). These individuals may have no warning symptoms and then suffer an untimely and premature death. We are certainly aware of the common risk factors for coronary artery disease, but many of these individuals have none. For some reason, these people experience a cardiac arrhythmia or irregular heart beat and collapse. If treated immediately with defibrillation– an electrical shock– the chances for survival are markedly increased.

WHAT IS SUDDEN CARDIAC ARREST? Sudden cardiac death occurs when the electrical system of the heart functions abnormally and a cardiac arrhythmia occurs. The most common arrhythmia is ventricular fibrillation, which is completely uncoordinated beating of the heart muscle. When this occurs, this fragmented movement of the heart does not pump blood adequately to the rest of the body and within a few minutes death ensues.

WHAT ARE THE WARNING SIGNS FOR SCA? In more than one-half of all cases, there are no warning signs and symptoms. It is well known that coronary artery disease may present itself with symptoms of chest pain, shortness of breath, nausea, vomiting, abdominal pain, sweating, arm pain or jaw pain, just to name a few. So when an individual experiences these problems, they must seek immediate medical attention, as SCA may be imminent.

WHAT IS THE TREATMENT FOR SCA? Since the electrical system of the heart is disrupted, the immediate treatment is rapid defibrillation. This is electrical shocking of the heart, which is accomplished with an AED. An electrical charge is then delivered to reset the natural pacemaker of the heart. Many times, only one shock is required. The amount of energy delivered ranges from 70 to 360 Joules.

Recent medical literature has shown that if defibrillation occurs within a couple of minutes, the success of survival may be 80 percent. It has also been shown that the chances of survival decrease about 10 percent with each minute that passes and after about 10 minutes, the chance of survival is 0 percent with no defibrillation. Thus, immediate defibrillation yields the greatest chance for success of surviving SCA. Nationally it has been shown that over the years, the chances of surviving an out-of-hospital cardiac arrest are only 5 percent! This can be improved with the public use of AEDs.

CARDIORESPIRATORY

ARE AEDS EASY TO USE?   Yes. The technology has improved over the years and the device is small and training is minimal.   Basically, the AED is a small laptop computer that delivers a charge of electricity through patches that are attached to the human body, one over the chest and one on the back.

The patches are placed on the body and the computer interprets the heart rhythm. If the heart rhythm requires an electrical charge to be delivered, the AED voice prompts the operator to press the button to deliver the shock. After the shock is delivered, the heart rhythm is re-assessed and another shock may be required. The AED tells the operator what to do and does not allow a normal beating heart to be shocked.

WHAT TRAINING IS REQUIRED?   At present, many states have public access defibrillation laws that dictate the use of AEDs. The American Heart Association and the American Red Cross offer half-day training courses in the assessment and treatment of SCA and the use of the AED. Cardiopulmonary Resuscitation (CPR) training may be included in the program.

WHAT IS THE COST OF AN AED?   Depending on the device, prices may range from $1500-$3000 per AED. The cost depends on the features present, accessories, and the number of AEDs purchased. In developing an AED program for your community, it is important to align agencies so there is no duplication of service and a seamless program can be formed and delivered.

WHAT ELSE CAN I DO?   The success of public assess defibrillation has been proven around the country. It is essential that the program continue to expand in all communities. This should be accomplished through local government authorities, private industry and business. A concerted effort through community leaders and private citizens can ensure a strong public access defibrillation program that will prevent premature death.

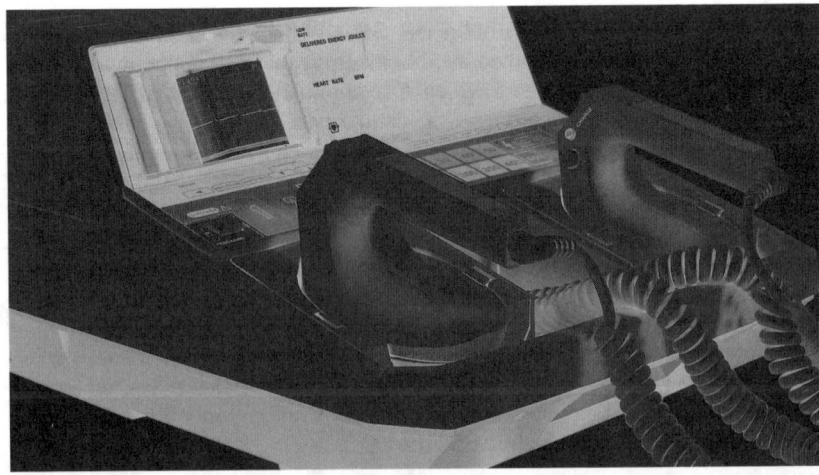

coronary artery bypass grafting (CABG)

Former President Bill Clinton underwent a coronary artery bypass grafting (CABG) procedure. This procedure is one of the most aggressive approaches to treating heart disease and is advised for a select group of patients with significant heart disease who are also able to withstand the stress of the surgery.

Each year, about 350,000 patients undergo CABG with a mortality rate of 3 to 4 percent. Fortunately for President Clinton, CABG has a proven track record of success and safety.

WHAT IS CORONARY ARTERY DISEASE? The heart is a muscle that requires blood supply. Exercise and activity will cause a demand for an increased blood flow to the heart muscle. When the blood vessels are narrowed with a plaque, inadequate blood flow is provided to the muscle. As a result, a person may experience chest pain or an aching feeling. A variety of other symptoms may be present including nausea, vomiting, sweating, jaw pain, arm pain and shortness of breath. This may be an indication of decreased blood supply to the heart, due to the narrowed arteries.

The narrowing of the arteries will occur over years. The well-known risk factors that lead to the narrowing include smoking, high blood pressure, high cholesterol, diabetes and family history. Many of these risk factors can be controlled to decrease the risk of developing coronary artery disease.

HOW IS THIS DIAGNOSED? When a patient experiences chest pain and shortness of breath, as in the case of Clinton, a medical workup is required. This includes an electrocardiogram (EKG), blood tests, possible stress test and coronary angiography. Coronary angiography, or catheterization, injects dye into the heart vessels as they are x-rayed. This test actually shows the architecture of vessels and if they are narrowed. A narrowed vessel of 50 to 70 percent may produce symptoms. A single narrowed vessel may be opened with a balloon, but if several vessels are involved, balloon angioplasty may not be safe or curative. Then, CABG is recommended.

WHAT IS CABG? In order to improve blood supply to the heart muscle, the narrowed portion of the coronary artery must be bypassed. A healthy artery or vein taken from the chest wall, arm or leg is attached above the narrowing and

CARDIORESPIRATORY

then attached to a vessel below the narrowing. This allows an adequate blood supply to be provided below the blocked artery.

A cardiothoracic surgeon will perform the operation. A cardiologist performs the catheterization prior to the surgery and helps the heart surgeon manage the patient medically in the hospital. The surgical procedure usually takes about four hours and a patient may be hospitalized for about five days. It is interesting to note that the heart is actually stopped while the doctors work on the heart and the patient's life is sustained by the heart-lung machine.

WHAT ARE THE RISKS? CABG is one of the most common major surgical operations performed in the United States today. The mortality rate from the procedure is about 3 to 4 percent. Exposure to anesthesia is a risk and exposure time should always be minimized. There is a small risk of stroke that can occur during the surgery.

In the post-operative period, a patient may develop bleeding at the surgical sites. There is a possibility of infection at the surgical site. Pneumonia may develop since the patient has been placed on a breathing machine and it may be difficult to breath after the surgery. In addition, there is a risk of the grafts blocking and they may need to be replaced.

Some other post-operative complications may involve the heart developing an arrhythmia or irregular heart beat. Many patients develop atrial fibrillation. Most of these problems can be treated with additional medications.

WHAT HAPPENS AFTER SURGERY? Most patients are hospitalized for about five days. Activities are slowly increased and cardiac rehabilitation is started. This is a very important aspect of the recovery period and must be continued for several weeks after the procedure. The patient must alter their life style in order to ensure success and a long, healthy life. In general, a patient such as former President Clinton, can be expected to have an uneventful recovery and experience a normal life span. His medical condition will be closely monitored by his physicians for the rest of his life, as it is with all CABG patients.

emphysema

No matter what generation you belonged to, everyone knew the "King of Late Night." The recent death of Johnny Carson has been attributed to emphysema, a common lung condition that is almost exclusively caused by smoking. A large percentage of the people who are afflicted could have prevented its development through smoking cessation.

WHAT IS EMPHYSEMA? Emphysema is one of the most severe forms of lung disease. Chronic Obstructive Pulmonary Disease (COPD) is a broader category of lung diseases that includes emphysema, which is usually an end-stage disease process. Other forms of associated lung diseases include chronic bronchitis and asthma.

With emphysema, the tiny air sacs at the end of the bronchial tube become damaged and over-inflated. When these tiny air sacs, known as alveoli, are damaged, it becomes harder and harder to breath. Patients that are affected have a cough and shortness of breath.

In the United States, over 16 million people suffer from COPD. Of these 16 million people, over 2 million suffer from emphysema and about 1,100 people die each year from this disease. Unfortunately, Johnny Carson was one of these statistics.

WHAT CAUSES EMPHYSEMA? Smoking causes over 80 percent of all cases of emphysema. A small percentage of cases are due to a hereditary condition whereby the lung does not produce a protein within the lung. This is a very rare condition. Other causes include exposure to pollution and second-hand smoke. Medical literature continues to support the danger of second-hand smoke leading to the development of many lung diseases.

Chronic exposure to smoke damages the elastic fibers in the lung and the tiny air sacs. Smoke also paralyzes the little hairs, called cilia, that help keep the air passages clean. Smoke interferes with the sweeping action of these little hairs and irritants remain in the lungs. This eventually causes inflammation of the bronchial tubes and breakdown of the elasticity of the lungs. The alveoli are the interface between inhaled oxygen and the blood stream. When damaged, this alters the body's ability to obtain oxygen and leads to breathlessness.

WHAT ARE THE SYMPTOMS? Patients with emphysema most commonly feel short of breath. This may start as shortness of breath with significant activity and progress to severe shortness of breath while at rest. Some patients have shortness of breath even while lying down. Other symptoms include a progressive cough. This may start as a morning cough and progress to a constant cough.

As the disease progresses, the work of breathing leads to fatigue. Patients may be too tired to eat and start to lose weight. This is a vicious cycle. The emphysema can get so bad that the patient cannot eat because they cannot catch their breath during chewing.

WHAT IS THE TREATMENT? Stopping smoking and exposure to irritants can reverse the early stages of COPD. Once a person suffers from emphysema, which is late in the disease process, reversal cannot occur. Regardless, smoking cessation will improve the quality of life of an affected patient.

Once the diagnosis is made on the basis of history, physical examination and chest x-ray, medications can be prescribed to help with breathing. Albuterol is a medicine that enlarges the bronchioles and allows for greater air passage. There are numerous other inhalers that are similar to albuterol that can be prescribed as well.

Steroids, which decrease inflammation, can also be prescribed. They may be in the form of oral prednisone or in an inhaled form. Both are very effective in helping improve the breathing process and decreasing inflammation of the bronchiole tubes.

Lastly, patients with emphysema may experience more frequent episodes of bronchitis. The increased sputum production may become infected requiring the use of antibiotics.

WHAT ELSE CAN BE DONE? Most importantly, smoking cessation is essential in preventing the development of emphysema. A healthy life style is important and the avoidance of second-hand smoke is important. In the event that you feel that you need help with these issues, seek medical attention. You may be improving your chances of living a little longer.

sudden cardiac death (SCD)

The death of San Francisco 49ers guard, Thomas Herrion, raised our awareness of sudden death in athletes. The autopsy report from the Denver coroner has thus proved inconclusive, but the results of toxicology and drug tests are currently pending.

Let's look a little more closely at sudden death in athletes. We will review the causes and the screening techniques that should be implemented.

HOW COMMON ARE SUDDEN DEATHS IN ATHLETES? These types of deaths date back to 490 BC when, according to legend, a Greek messenger ran a 26.2-mile marathon and dropped dead at the finish line.

A variety of statistics have shown that the chance of sudden death in an apparently healthy athlete ranges from 1 in 200,000 athletes to 1 in 750,000 athletes. Fortunately, this problem is not too common.

WHAT ARE THE CAUSES? The leading cause of sudden death in an athlete is due to heart disease. Usually, in younger athletes, a birth defect or congenital problem is the primary cause. In older athletes, acquired diseases such as vascular disease are the cause.

Some conditions known to cause sudden cardiac death include hypertrophic cardiomyopathy, which is a genetic condition. The heart muscle is enlarged leading to smaller chambers in the heart. This abnormality in the muscle fibers leads to problems with the electrical system. Patients with these problems have a higher incidence of occurrence of cardiac arrhythmias. This is usually a silent problem until the athlete dies.

Other causes of sudden death in athletes have been shown to be secondary to acquired problems such as narrowing in the arteries leading to a blockage that causes a heart attack or myocardial infarction. Sometimes, there are congenital problems in how the vessels on the heart muscle are arranged. Also, some people are genetically predisposed to developing coronary artery disease and high cholesterol.

It has also been found that certain infections can cause an inflammation of the heart muscle, thus leading to irregular beats. Some viruses may infect the heart and lead to temporary or permanent damage.

HOW DOES ONE SCREEN FOR SUDDEN CARDIAC DEATH?

This is a very frustrating problem for health care providers, as it is like searching for a needle in the haystack. A risk analysis must be done to determine who requires more comprehensive screening. It is important to remember that this is not a very common problem and it would be too costly to screen every single athlete with aggressive testing.

Those at risk for sudden cardiac death are athletes with a family history of sudden death or early heart disease. When athletes experience unprovoked fainting, concern should be raised. Other medical conditions include those with Marfan's syndrome, which is a genetic problem in really tall athletes. When there are valve problems in the heart, there are risks of heart beat irregularities. It is also important to remember that drug abuse is a leading cause of heart problems in this patient population.

WHAT ELSE SHOULD BE DONE? Young athletes should be screened for health problems. The standard athletic physical is a good place to start. The health care provider will assess risks and determine if further testing is required. This may include echocardiography, which is an ultrasound picture of the heart structure, and screening for drugs and alcohol.

Other medical conditions may be identified during this examination that may place the athlete at risk. It has been shown that sudden deaths are higher in college-aged males who participate in football or basketball, but no athlete is immune.

Most importantly, it should be remembered that this is not a very common problem and you should not worry about your son or daughter participating in athletics at the elementary, high school or collegiate level, as long as they are appropriately assessed prior to participation.

tracheostomy

Pope John Paul II, once a vibrant and active man, continued to deteriorate, suffering from the effects of Parkinson's disease and was later hospitalized with influenza and respiratory difficulties. Then, about a week after discharge from Rome's Gimelli Hospital, the Pope was rushed back for the treatment of acute respiratory distress. Part of the treatment program involved the surgical placement of a tracheostomy. This is a fairly common surgical procedure and many patients live long healthy lives with a tracheostomy.

WHAT IS A TRACHEOSTOMY? A tracheostomy (trach) is a surgical procedure that places an opening in the neck below the larynx or Adam's apple. This surgical opening allows for more direct passage of oxygen into the lungs. Once the opening is made, a small tube is placed inside in order to keep the hole open.

There are temporary and permanent tracheostomies. The temporary trach is used to bypass an upper airway obstruction for a brief period of time, to allow for healing. The permanent trach is used in cases when permanent bypass is necessary, in cases of cancer, for example.

WHY IS A TRACH PLACED? There are numerous reasons why a trach may be placed. In the emergency department, the procedure may be performed to open a difficult airway. This may be used in cases of facial trauma or acute upper airway infection. This is a not a very common emergency procedure, because as emergency physicians, we have numerous other ways to secure an airway.

In the case of the Pope, this procedure was completed in a more elective fashion. One might assume that he had difficulty in keeping his airway clear due to the muscle weakness caused by his Parkinson's disease. His posture had deteriorated and this may have contributed to the inability to keep the airway open. Of course, this is all speculation, as release of information has been guarded by the Vatican.

In general, clinical indications for the placement of the trach are to address birth defects in the airway, severe trauma or disfigurement. There may be cancer blocking the airway, that may be removed or bypassed. As with the Pope, there may be paralysis of the muscles that affect swallowing due to a medical condition. Lastly, patients that are on a respirator for a long period of time may need a trach, as the tube in the lungs may lead to complications in the upper airway.

WHAT ARE THE RISKS WITH THE PROCEDURE? As with any surgical procedure, a patient is at risk for developing an infection in the post-operative period at the actual surgical site or in the lungs (pneumonia). There is also a risk of bleeding or problems with breathing. Long-term complications may involve the development of scar tissue at the site.

WHAT HAPPENS AFTER SURGERY? In general, the procedure takes about one-half hour and is completed in the operating room, usually by a physician specializing in the ear, nose, and throat. The post-operative recovery may last one to three days.

The patient will need to adjust to breathing through the tube in the neck. There will be a training period necessary to learn how to live with this tube and how to speak. Special care of the area is also important.

Most patients who undergo this procedure will adapt quite quickly and lead a fairly normal life. Support groups are available to assist the patient and family with this new medical condition. Patients will have to adhere to some special precautions to protect this open airway from water, dust, powder and other irritants. Overall, keeping the area clean will be essential to the long-term health of the patient.

women
& CHD

February has been designated as the month for awareness of heart disease in women. The "Red Dress" campaign has been launched to make everyone aware of the seriousness of heart disease in women. Over the years, it has been thought that mostly men suffered heart attacks and died. This is not true and the American Heart Association has just launched a campaign to heighten the awareness of the problem of coronary heart disease (CHD) in women. In addition, evidence-based guidelines have been released showing the effectiveness of factors that can be modified, thereby improving longevity.

HOW SERIOUS IS THIS PROBLEM? CHD is the leading cause of death of women in the United States today. About a half million women succumb to cardiovascular disease each year. The second leading cause of death is cancer and then stroke, which has similar risk factors to CHD. It is interesting to note that twice as many women die from a heart attack as opposed to cancer.

In addition, there are over 8 million women in the United States living with some form of heart disease and more women than men will die from heart disease.

WHAT ARE RISK FACTORS FOR CHD IN WOMEN? The risk factors of CHD for women are the same as in men, but the presentation of symptoms can be different. The major risk factors for developing heart trouble include smoking, high cholesterol, obesity, high blood pressure, diabetes, inactivity and family history of premature heart disease. Most of the risk factors can be modified to improve one's chance of not suffering a heart attack.

The American Heart Association has just released several guidelines. Hundreds of articles and medical studies were reviewed and their recommendations are based on medical fact. These recommendations are shown to improve one's chance of not suffering a heart attack. Additionally, therapies are recommended for those that have been afflicted with heart disease in order to improve the quality of life and extend one's life.

WHAT ARE THE SYMPTOMS OF A HEART ATTACK? It is well known that heart disease can present with many different symptoms such as chest pain, shortness of breath, arm pain, nausea, vomiting and sweating. In

CARDIORESPIRATORY

women, the symptoms are not always as clear-cut and may fool the health care provider. Signs of CHD may include abdominal pain, nausea, "heart burn," weakness or just not feeling "right."

An evaluation by a health care provider is important when any of the symptoms are present. Your provider will need to take all of the pieces of the clinical puzzle and put them together in order to render appropriate treatment.

WHAT ARE THE RECOMMENDATIONS? It has been shown that quitting smoking will decrease the chances of developing CHD. This will also improve one's chances of not developing cancer or lung disease.

Elevated cholesterol must be treated through a variety of therapies including diet, exercise and medication. This is essential in preventing the development of CHD whereby the cholesterol deposits in the coronary arteries, causing narrowing.

The management of high blood pressure is important. Prolonged periods of high blood pressure have been shown to damage the arteries and stretch out the heart muscle. In addition, one is placed at risk for the development of stroke and congestive heart failure, which is a weakened, ineffective pumping heart.

In the presence of heart disease, certain medications have been proven effective. Aspirin is one of the most cost-effective drugs on the market today and it has significant impact on women's heart disease. Daily aspirin administration should only come as a directive from your health care provider. Other medications used after a heart attack include beta-blockers. The use of estrogen and progestin was originally thought to protect against CHD, but those recommendations are being re-evaluated.

WHAT SHOULD I DO? It is important to realize that women are at significant risk for heart disease including heart attack and death. Health care providers must consider heart disease when women present with suspicious symptoms, especially accompanied by risk factors. Lastly, it is essential that you take the recommendations seriously and modify many of the risk factors that can lead to coronary artery disease and premature death.

appendicitis

Appendicitis: More Than Just a Tummy Ache.

Appendicitis can affect all age groups, but it is more unusual in the very young and the elderly. In the elderly, there is an increased chance of complications. Because of this, it is important that the physician test for other conditions before diagnosing appendicitis.

In the young, left-sided abdominal pain is usually constipation. A pediatric enema in the ER usually cures the problem. In the adult population, left sided abdominal pain may be diverticulitis or a kidney stone.

WHAT IS APPENDICITIS? Appendicitis is a "flaring up" or inflammation of the appendix, a small outgrowth of the small intestine located in the lower right area of the abdomen. The appendix serves no major function, but it can become blocked by food or inflammation. The inflammation causes swelling and blockage that causes pain.

WHAT ARE THE SYMPTOMS? Pain is the trademark symptom of appendicitis, usually accompanied by nausea and loss of appetite. The pain may actually start out in the center of the abdomen, but it will settle in the lower right area. Strangely enough, if appendicitis is the affliction in question, the doctor will ask whether you experienced abdominal pain while riding in a bumpy car.

Symptoms can occur in the span of two hours to two days. Appendicitis can be very difficult for the doctor to diagnose. As a result, the doctor will review your history and perform a physical exam. Many times, the doctor will have the patient return for another exam within 12 to 24 hours, because the diagnosis is not always clear at first. Re-examination is very important in making a correct diagnosis.

WHAT TESTS CAN I EXPECT? Laboratory tests and x-rays may help in diagnosing appendicitis. A complete blood count may reveal a high white blood cell count, which is a sign of infection or inflammation. A urine test should be done to rule out a bladder infection or a kidney stone. A CAT scan, which is often used to locate kidney stones, can help in diagnosing appendicitis because the appendix can be seen on this scan as well. But even with all of this modern technology, diagnosing appendicitis can be very difficult. In fact, about 20 percent of appendixes that are removed are normal!

GASTRO-INTESTINAL

WHAT IS THE TREATMENT? Surgery is the only option to remove an inflamed and infected appendix. The procedure can be done through an open cut in the abdomen or through laproscopic surgery. Laproscopic surgery involves a few very small incisions, with the appendix being removed through a scope. This procedure lasts less than one-half hour, and the patient is usually discharged from the hospital on the same day, or the day after surgery. Patients may have some abdominal tenderness for a couple of days after the surgery. Complication rates are low, but can include a wound infection.

WHAT CAN I DO? Unfortunately, appendicitis cannot be prevented. If a patient has right lower abdominal pain, they need to be examined. Also, patients should not eat anything prior to coming to the hospital in the event that they do have appendicitis and surgery is needed. And since a urine test will usually be required, patients should not empty their bladder prior to coming in for an examination.

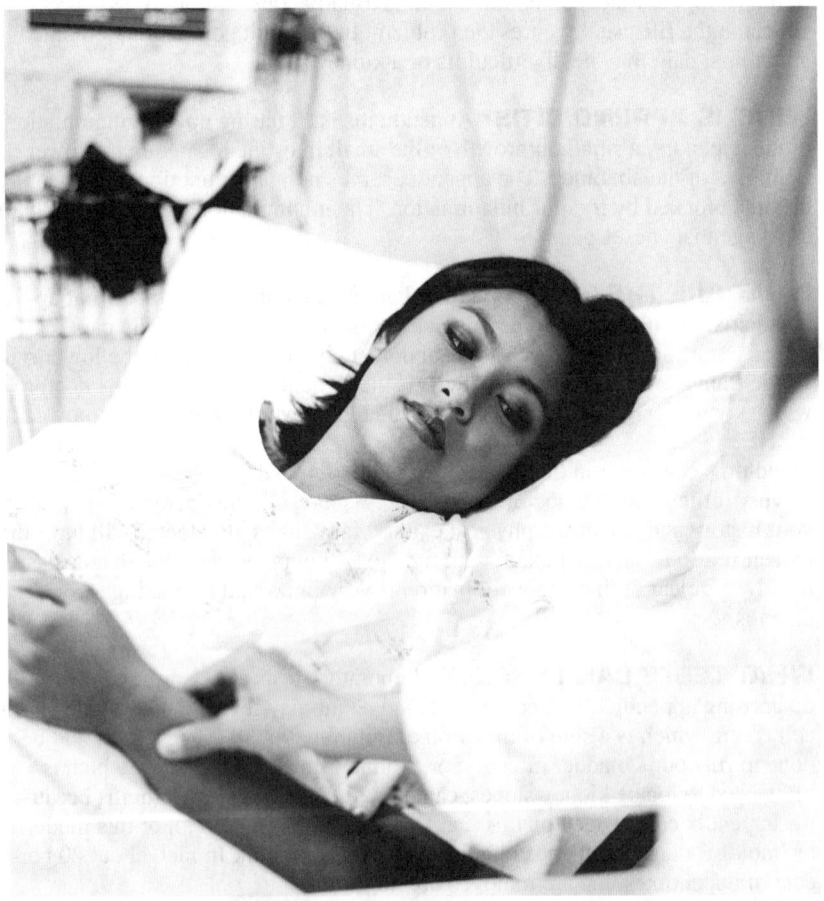

capsule endoscopy

As I travel around the country for business or pleasure, I usually remain in touch through wireless technology. Whether in a hotel, coffee shop or airport, it is great to be able to open your laptop and log on. Also, I usually have my digital camera in hand to capture important sites and moments.

Well, this technology is also important in medicine. Recently, new techniques have become available to evaluate the gastrointestinal (GI) tract using both wireless and digital photo technology. No, you do not have to swallow your laptop or your digital camera! You simply swallow a digital capsule the size of a vitamin pill.

WHAT IS WIRELESS CAPSULE ENDOSCOPY? In this procedure, a patient swallows a small disposable capsule that contains a digital camera that emits light. As the capsule goes through the GI system, it takes pictures of the entire system, from the mouth all the way down through the end of the colon.

About two images per second are taken over an eight-hour period and they are sent to a small recording device worn on the belt of a patient. The recorder is the size of a Walkman and it receives the images from electrodes (wires) that are taped to the skin. After eight hours, the recorder is removed and the pictures are retrieved and then studied by the doctor.

WHEN WAS THIS DEVELOPED? In 1981, an Israeli physician developed this unique and noninvasive concept. It took 20 years for the process to be refined and in 2001, the Givens M2A capsule was approved and released for use. M2A stands for mouth to anus. This noninvasive GI procedure is available at several centers around the country.

WHY IS THIS USED? Capsule endoscopy (CE) in another way for physicians to evaluate the GI tract. Conventional methods of study have included the barium x-ray study, CT scan or upper and lower endoscopy. The most common procedure today is the upper endoscopy and lower endoscopy procedures.

The upper procedure looks at the esophagus (food tube) and stomach, while the lower endoscopy or colonoscopy looks at the colon to the level of the cecum, near the appendix. But in these procedures, about 20 feet of small bowel is missed with the scope. This is where CE may be useful, but not a replacement, for conventional GI procedures.

GASTRO-INTESTINAL

The CE looks for causes of unexplained pain or discomfort in the GI tract. The procedure also helps to evaluate for bleeding, ulcers, polyps (benign growths) or cancerous tumors. Unfortunately, even though the procedure is very good, things can be missed.

WHAT IS THE PROCEDURE? The process is quite simple. The patient will not be able to eat after midnight, but no extensive bowel preparation is need. The digital disposable capsule pill is swallowed and shortly thereafter, pictures of the intestinal insides are recorded.

Even though CE may miss some abnormalities, it is an excellent screening tool. It may be hard to actually identify a specific location of the problem, but the information is still vital. In addition, it is essential that patients undergo conventional screening tests to assess the GI system.

WHAT ARE THE SIDE EFFECTS? No major side effects have been associated with CE. Some people have experienced bloating, gas and discomfort, but none of these effects are unusual. The biggest risk is an intestinal obstruction, especially if there is a narrowing in the intestine caused by a tumor.

WHAT SHOULD I DO? If you are suffering from stomach and intestinal problems, you need to be evaluated by your health care provider. If you are at risk for GI cancer, this tool may become one of the tests that may help with the screening process.

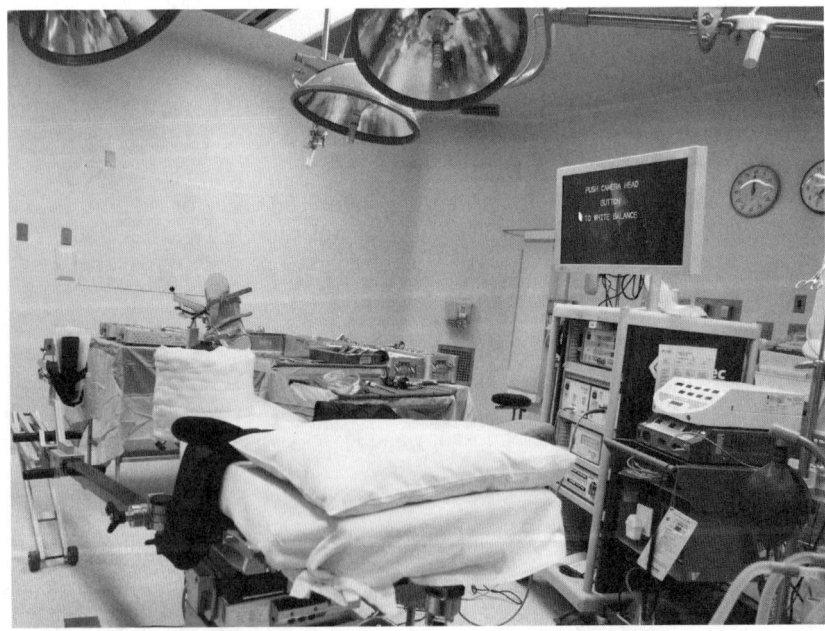

cholesterol

A recent study at the University of California-Los Angeles (UCLA) has shown that the use of a common class of cholesterol-lowering drug, a statin, can improve longevity in patients with congestive heart failure. These medications are used in people who suffer from heart disease and vascular disease, and studies continue to prove that these drugs help in prolonging life.

WHAT IS HIGH CHOLESTEROL? High cholesterol, also known as hypercholesterolemia, is a medical condition whereby a level of cholesterol in the blood is high. There are good and bad forms of cholesterol in the body. The body needs cholesterol in order to repair damaged cell membranes, develop and maintain nerve cells, as well as help in the production of hormones. Excessive amounts of cholesterol usually come from diet and the liver produces these levels during the breakdown of dietary fats, carbohydrates and proteins.

WHAT ARE THE TYPES OF CHOLESTEROL? The good cholesterol is called a high-density lipoproteins (HDL) and this one helps in keeping the artery walls clean and free from a buildup of the plaques that cause narrowing of the interior portion of the artery.

The bad cholesterol is called low-density lipoprotein (LDL) and it carries a great deal of cholesterol. The LDLs leave behind deposits in the arteries of the heart, that causes narrowing of these vessels. The narrowed vessels eventually lead to coronary artery disease and the possibility of a heart attack. Arteries in the brain and the extremities can be affected as well.

WHAT CAUSES ELEVATED CHOLESTEROL? A person develops high levels of cholesterol through a diet that is rich in fats and cholesterol. In addition, there is a hereditary factor that determines how the body processes cholesterol. Underlying diseases of the kidney, thyroid, liver and diabetes can also elevate blood levels.

WHAT ARE SYMPTOMS? There are no direct symptoms of hypercholesterolemia. The elevated states are usually diagnosed incidentally through routine physical examination, especially if there is a strong family history. Unfortunately, some people wait too long and the disease is diagnosed after a heart attack and the patient is hospitalized.

Other symptoms may present when the vessels in the legs are affected. For example, a person may develop severe pain after only walking a short distance. This may be an indication that the vessels are narrowed, not allowing adequate blood supply.

HOW IS IT DIAGNOSED? Elevated levels of cholesterol are found through a fasting blood test. Usually, a person will have to fast for 12 hours prior to a blood test. The blood test will look at the total cholesterol level, the level of the HDL, and the level of the LDL. In general, a total level of cholesterol under 200 mg/dl is good, along with an LDL level less than 130, and an HDL level of 45 or higher. These values are a range and you must discuss the results with your health care provider.

WHAT IS THE TREATMENT? Cholesterol-lowering guidelines and treatment will be recommended by your health care provider. Initially, diet, exercise and weight loss are recommended, prior to a commitment to expensive, long-term medications. It is important to modify your lifestyle including smoking cessation and moderation of alcohol intake.

When the conservative measures fail, medication may be necessary. There are a wide variety of cholesterol-lowering medications and each medicine has its merits. Your provider will need to determine which class of medication is best on the basis of several factors.

Today, statins are the most commonly prescribed cholesterol-lowering drugs and they have many proven long-term health benefits, impacting the heart, blood vessels, brain and bones.

WHAT ELSE CAN I DO? Prevention is always best and is essential to decrease your risk for coronary artery disease and stroke. Lowering your cholesterol levels can improve your quality of life and increase your life span. Maintain a healthy diet, exercise regularly, lose weight if necessary, stop smoking and monitor your cholesterol level each year.

diverticulitis

Abdominal pain is a common complaint seen in emergency departments on a daily basis, but is a concern that can be easily addressed by a health care provider through a simple evaluation to determine the specific cause.

Abdominal pain may be caused by a simple upset stomach, heartburn, appendicitis, bowel obstruction, kidney stone, urinary tract infection, ovarian cyst or diverticular disease. If the more serious concern of diverticular disease is diagnosed, then treatment should begin.

WHAT IS DIVERTICULAR DISEASE? Diverticula are little pouches in the large intestine that develop over years. These little pouches are actual herniations of weakened bowel that push from the inside of the intestine outward. The inside of the large intestine or colon should look nice and smooth. With diverticula, the colon looks like a cobblestone road with the pouches extending into the wall of the muscular intestine.

When a person has several diverticula, the diagnosis of diverticulosis is made. When stool and food particles get caught in these pouches, they become inflamed and infected. This is called diverticulitis. The older you become, the greater chance you have of developing diverticular disease.

HOW COMMON IS DIVERTICULOSIS? This is a very common cause of intestinal problems and the incidence clearly increases with age. At age 65, about 50 percent of all Americans have diverticulosis. That incidence will increase by another 15 percent at age 85. It is a little more common in women than men by about 10 percent. It is interesting to note that of all people with diverticulosis, up to 25 percent will develop a case of diverticulitis that will require medical or surgical management.

WHAT CAUSES DIVERTICULOSIS? In the early 1900s, diverticular disease was first diagnosed in the United States. The American diet of processed foods that lack in fiber has lead to a steady increase in the disease. Constipation is felt to be a leading irritant whereby the increased pressure of stool in the colon leads to a weakening of the wall of the intestine. The weakening of the intestinal wall leads to the development of diverticula.

WHAT CAUSES DIVERTICULITIS? A person who has diverticulosis is at risk for developing inflammation and infection of the little pouches. These pouches retain bacteria, stool, and food leading to an irritated condition that requires medical and sometimes surgical management.

WHAT ARE THE SYMPTOMS OF DIVERTICULITIS? Most commonly, patients may present with vague complaints of abdominal pain. The pain is usually on the left side of the lower abdomen. It may be a rather sudden onset. The pain will worsen over time and may include nausea with vomiting. As the condition worsens, a person may develop a fever and become very ill. Left untreated, the pouches may become very inflamed and infected leading to rupture. This is a very serious condition and at this point, intestinal contents can spill inside the abdominal cavity, leading to a very serious infection.

HOW IS THIS DIAGNOSED? Many people know that they have diverticulosis, as it was incidentally diagnosed on a screening colon exam. But sometimes the presentation of abdominal pain is the first hint of a problem. The examining provider will get a history and perform a physical examination. Blood tests may point to inflammation or infection. The x-ray of choice is the CT scan, which looks at the structure of the intestine and whether an infection is present. An abscess or collection of pus may be seen in the most severe cases.

WHAT IS THE TREATMENT? Once the diagnosis is made, changes in diet to avoid seeds and grains are recommended. Bowel rest is important. In patients that have a mild case, a two-week course of oral antibiotics is recommended. In more serious cases, hospitalization is necessary to provide intravenous antibiotics. The most serious cases may require surgery to remove an abscess or a portion of the damaged colon.

WHAT ELSE CAN I DO? Prevention is key, especially once the diagnosis of diverticulosis is made. The avoidance of foods with seeds, grains and vegetables difficult to digest is essential. It is very important to seek medical attention when you develop abdominal pain, as diverticular disease is only one possible diagnosis out of many others.

food bolus

During the holiday season, invitations to cocktail socials, holiday dinners and company parties fill our mailboxes. Our social calendars fill, as well as our stomachs. At the hospital, we start to see an increase of patients that may suffer the effects of all of these events. One of the common problems that occurs during this time of the year is the Steakhouse Syndrome, known in the medical world as esophageal food bolus (EFB) or impaction.

WHAT IS STEAKHOUSE SYNDROME? The Steakhouse Syndrome, or EFB, is named after a condition that occurs when people are usually eating meat, drinking alcohol, inadequately chewing their food and then swallowing a large piece of meat. The meat then gets stuck in the lower esophagus, which is just above the opening of the stomach. As a result, no food or liquid may pass this blockage. There may be fairly intense pain and the patient may think that they are having a heart attack. They may be unable to control liquids and secretions, which can result in fits of coughing and choking.

WHO IS AFFECTED? A majority of patients that initially present with EFB are adults that are in their 40s and 50s. This is a very uncommon problem in children. It has been shown that 75 to 100 percent of those affected have an underlying problem in their esophagus. Those problems include a narrowing of the esophagus called a Schatzki's ring, esophageal stricture or spasm. It is important to remember that esophageal cancers do not usually present initially with a food bolus. So, if you are affected, do not worry that you have cancer!

WHAT ARE THE CAUSES? There are two reasons why an EFB develops. The initial problem involves the size of the piece of food trying to be ingested. Inadequate chewing will send a large piece food, usually meat, down to an opening that is too small and the meat gets stuck. Alcohol can be a factor leading to inadequate chewing, as well as the presence of dentures. Sometimes, people are embarrassed to spit out a large, tough piece of meat and attempt to swallow it. This leads to blockage of the esophagus.

Narrowing of the esophagus has numerous causes such as the Schatzki's ring, which may be a congenital problem. Other causes of esophageal narrowing may be secondary to years of reflux disease or heartburn. Caustic stomach contents splashing back up onto the esophageal tissue leads to chronic damage and scarring. This eventually narrows the opening into the stomach. Lastly, the esophagus may be damaged by drinking caustic substances in an attempt to kill one's self. Those who survive may have severe scarring and narrowing that can be a lifelong problem.

WHAT SHOULD I DO? In the event that you experience a food bolus, do not panic! Over three-fourths of these impactions will pass on their own. You may experience severe chest pain and start to salivate. If the food is not passing, you will need to come to the emergency department for treatment.

At the hospital, a simple diagnostic test involves drinking a small glass of water. If the esophagus is blocked, the water will not pass and further treatment will be provided. A diabetes medication called glucagon, has been shown to relax muscles and may allow for passage of the food. When this does not work, a physician specializing in endoscopy will be called to help. At this time, the patient will be sedated and a fiber optic scope will be passed down the esophagus and the food will be pushed into the stomach. Additionally, the physician will be able to look at the condition of the stomach and esophagus during the procedure.

WHAT IS THE FOLLOW-UP? It is important to identify the cause for the narrowing of the esophagus and have treatment provided. Schatzki's rings can be electively dilated or enlarged through another endoscopy procedure. Prevention of heartburn or reflux is essential through alterations in diet, eating habits and medications. The most common medications used are the H2 blockers or proton pump inhibitor medications. Both of these medications are in prescription and over-the-counter forms.

Overall, this is a fairly common problem. It is important to chew food appropriately and avoid excessive amounts of alcohol while dining. Seek medical attention if you have a food bolus and be sure to receive follow-up medical attention to prevent a reoccurrence.

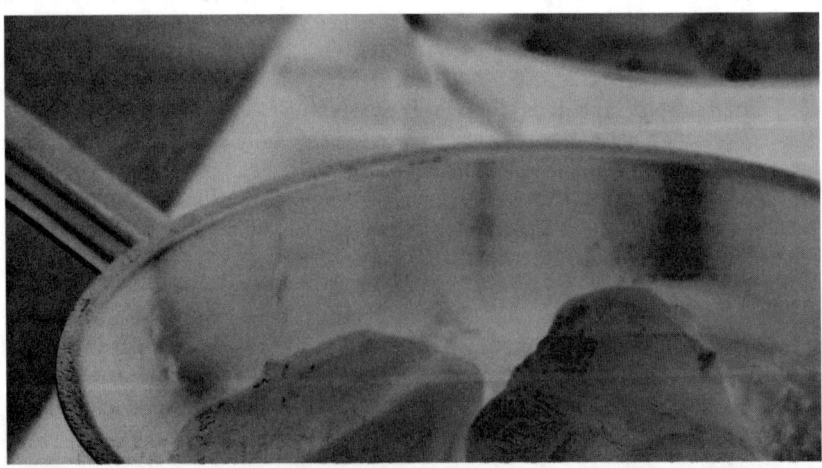

food poisoning

Are you getting bombarded with those department store flyers, attempting to catch your eye with sales on the latest and greatest outdoor grills? Because before you invest in a grill, it's important that you educate yourself on the safety of handling and grilling food for your summer parties. One outbreak of food poisoning, such as salmonella, is a sure way to have your guest list cut in half at your next gathering. So clean off those grills, prepare the marinade sauce, and get ready for a healthy summer of safe grilling!

WHAT IS FOOD POISONING? Food poisoning is a gastrointestinal (GI) illness that we develop after eating contaminated or improperly cooked food. The symptoms may be short-lived and are generally not life threatening, just very unpleasant.

WHAT CAUSES FOOD POISONING? Bacteria, viruses or a parasite may cause food poisoning. On a daily basis, we are all exposed to several of the above toxins in small amounts. We even ingest these bugs in small amounts. But when large amounts of a bacteria, viruses or parasites are ingested, symptoms and illness may occur.

Some of the common bacteria include staphylococcus and salmonella. Staphylococcus bacteria are the most common cause of food poisoning in the United States, followed by salmonella. Less common bacteria may include clostridium or bacillus. These bacteria, through improper handling or cooking, may contaminate foods. The food handler may be ill or the utensils used may be contaminated causing the bacteria to be transmitted to the food.

Most viruses that infect the human GI tract live in water. Drinking contaminated water or washing food with this water may infect humans. Additionally, seafood may also become infected from its contaminated environment.

Parasites are a little less common, but most people are familiar with trichinosis. This comes from the digestion of improperly cooked pork.

WHAT ARE THE SYMPTOMS? In general, the onset of symptoms may occur within an hour to several hours after the exposure to contaminated foods. Patients may complain of nausea, vomiting, abdominal cramping and diarrhea. The symptoms are brought on by the production of toxins from the offending bacteria or virus.

GASTRO-INTESTINAL

Food poisoning that is caused by staphylococcus may generate symptoms within 30 minutes of ingestion and may last for a day or two. Salmonella food poisoning generally has a longer onset of action and the course may last up to five days. The symptoms caused by both bacteria are almost the same, so one cannot differentiate the bacteria on the basis of symptoms.

The symptoms are usually self-limited and will resolve with symptomatic home treatments within a day or two. In the event that there is localized abdominal pain or fever, you must see your health care provider.

WHAT SHOULD I DO? As noted, there is no specific treatment for food poisoning. You may not feel like eating for a day or two, but it is important to remember that clear liquids can help in the healing process. You should also try to avoid all dairy products for a couple of days, as this may irritate your stomach. In the event that the above simple remedies do not help, you may need to see your doctor.

HOW IS IT DIAGNOSED? Usually, your health care provider will take a very accurate history, but it is important for you to confirm if others have the same exposure and symptoms. A culture of the stool may be obtained with prolonged cases and an antibiotic may be prescribed on the basis of these results. Anti-nauseant medications may be prescribed in order for the patient to orally rehydrate him or herself. Inpatient hospitalization is usually not required for treatment.

HOW CAN I PREVENT THIS? As you move outside to cook and dine, it is important to follow some simple rules. Be sure that all foods are appropriately stored in a cool environment until ready for cooking. Be sure to wash platters that have had the uncooked meats on them prior to serving the finished product. Make sure that your hands and utensils are washed after handling uncooked meats. Be sure to check on and follow temperature and time recommendations for grilling of meats. All of these recommendations require good common sense.

SHOULD I SEEK MEDICAL ATTENTION? Food poisoning is usually not life threatening and usually the remedies recommended above will take care of the situation. People at risk for complications are the very young and very old. Also, people with several underlying medical conditions or that have poor immune systems may require more aggressive treatment. As always, in the event that you are unsure about what to do, seek medical advice from a qualified health care professional.

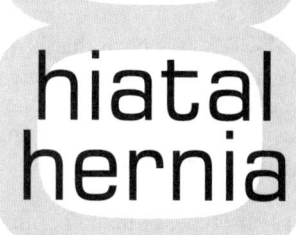

hiatal hernia

Each day in the emergency department, it is common for several patients to present with complaints of abdominal pain and chest pain. Many workups conclude that the pain is coming from the gastrointestinal (GI) tract because of gastro-esophageal reflux or heartburn. Reflux may be due to a structural abnormality called a hiatal hernia.

WHAT IS A HIATAL HERNIA? This medical condition is when part of the stomach comes through the hiatus– the hole in the diaphragm where the esophagus passes. The diaphragm is a very thin-walled muscle that separates the chest cavity from the abdominal cavity. The purpose of the diaphragm is to help with the process of breathing. Small hernias are quite common and go undiagnosed for a lifetime. The larger ones lead to more GI symptoms.

WHAT ARE THE SYMPTOMS? As noted, many people with a hiatal hernia never have symptoms and do not require treatment. But as the condition worsens and age increases, a person may feel the effects of the problem. The most common problems is "heartburn," where the digestive juices come up into the esophagus leading to a sour taste in the mouth. Many patients will notice that they have increased belching or vomiting.

Sometimes these symptoms may mimic a problem like heart disease. A person may think they are having a heart attack, because they have chest pain. They may also have some difficulty in swallowing or feel like the esophagus is blocked.

WHO IS AFFECTED? In the United States, this is a fairly common problem with a variety of presentations. About 10 percent of the patients with a hiatal hernia under the age of 40 and 70 percent of the patients are over 70.

More women than men have the condition, perhaps due to the intra-abdominal pressure and changes that are exerted from pregnancy. In the Western world, a fiber-depleted diet may also lead to an increase in frequency compared to our international associates.

WHAT ARE THE CAUSES? It is clear that increased age leads to development of a hiatal hernia. As the diaphragm muscle weakens, the esophagus is able to slide up into the chest cavity. Any time there is increased pressure in the abdominal cavity, as with straining or coughing, the esophagus may migrate upward. This is sometimes called a sliding hernia.

Another form, and more severe type, of hiatal hernia is the paraesophageal hernia. The opening in the diaphragm is much larger and part of the stomach may come into the chest cavity. There may be a twisting action of the stomach referred to as a rolling hernia.

HOW IS THIS DIAGNOSED? Many times a person may not have complaints and the condition is diagnosed during a search for another problem. But if a person is experiencing complaints of reflux, an upper GI x-ray or an upper endoscopy may make the diagnosis. These procedures will be ordered after your health care provider has taken a comprehensive history of symptoms and completed a physical examination. Laboratory studies, such as a blood test, will not aid in the diagnosis.

WHAT IS THE TREATMENT? When a person has symptoms, several treatment options will be prescribed. First, a change in lifestyle will be recommended including weight loss and a change in diet. A dietary log may be used to assess when the symptoms occur.

Some effective medicines include Maalox, H2 blockers such as Zantac and proton pump inhibitors such as Prilosec. These types of medications are available over-the-counter and in prescribed form.

With severe and refractory cases, a surgical procedure may be recommended. This is after the conservative treatment measures have failed. More recently, a laparoscopic procedure has been perfected. The laparoscopic procedure is less invasive and involves much smaller incisions. There is less of risk of complications such as bleeding and scarring. If you require surgery, be sure to have a surgeon well-trained in the procedure performing the operation.

irritable bowel syndrome (IBS)

During the holiday season, we may start to experience some stomach discomfort and change in bowel habits. There may be some pain, bloating and diarrhea. This may be due to a change in eating habits, yet it could be a more a chronic problem. Your health care provider may diagnose you with Irritable Bowel Syndrome (IBS).

WHAT IS IRRITABLE BOWEL SYNDROME? IBS is a disorder of the colon that involves digestion and proper functioning of the bowels. Primarily, there is abnormal motility of the colon, with either low or excessive movements of the colon.

It is important to note that IBS is not a disease and there are no structural abnormalities that can be identified on physical exam, radiographic testing or laboratory testing. This is purely a functional digestive disorder that is related to the motility of the intestines.

WHAT ARE THE SYMPTOMS? The symptoms of IBS are very nonspecific and range from abdominal pain, cramping, spasms, bloating, gas and bouts of diarrhea followed by bouts of constipation.

The main hallmark of the disorder is the sudden onset of diarrhea that may be followed by constipation. Patients may eventually pass only mucous in their bowel movements. Irritants may include large meals and stress that lead to pain and bloating. Certain foods, beverages, and medications may be irritating factors as well.

The syndrome and the symptoms can be quite bothersome and painful. It is important to remember that there is no structural damage that is occurring during the presentation of the symptoms. IBS does not make one more susceptible to cancer or any other more serious diseases. Most importantly, bleeding and weight loss are not consistent with IBS and those symptoms must be thoroughly investigated!

WHO IS AFFECTED? In the United States, one in five Americans has IBS. This is the most common digestive disorder diagnosed by health care providers. The incidence is more prevalent in women. The age of onset is usually in the late teens to early 20s.

WHAT IS THE CAUSE? Researchers and physicians have not identified a specific cause of IBS and it appears that it is not related to one specific factor. It does appear that patients with IBS are much more sensitive to stress and different foods.

It has been shown that those who suffer from IBS have no physical abnormality of the colon. The motility is affected during temporary periods. It can occur in waves of spasms and then the movement of the intestines stop, leading to constipation. The rapid movement of the colon does not allow for proper absorption of food leading to diarrhea. Conversely, the slowing of the colon leads to constipation.

HOW IS IT DIAGNOSED? IBS is a diagnosis of exclusion meaning that all other physical and psychological causes of the disorder must be ruled out prior to defining a condition as IBS.

A careful history and physical examination must be completed documenting gastrointestinal history and habits. Appropriate laboratory studies will be completed and x-rays may be necessary. Eventually, it may be determined that a flexible sigmoidoscopy or colonoscopy will be necessary to look at the inside integrity of the intestines.

If all testing is negative, then the diagnosis of IBS will be made. Specific criterions are used and they include abdominal pain for a total of 12 weeks each year. This does not mean constant pain for this time period. The patient must also experience relief of pain from a bowel movement, pain with varied frequency of stools or a change in stool consistency.

WHAT IS THE TREATMENT? Several physical and psychological treatments have been known to be successful. There are some antimotility medications that may slow the colon. Constipation may need to be treated as well. Recently, hypnotherapy and other forms of psychotherapy have been shown to work.

It is essential that the proper diagnosis be made prior to instituting any therapy. Your health care provider must rule out any serious disease prior to improving the disorder and it important that you seek treatment if you are bothered by these symptoms.

pancreatitis

John Ashcroft, the former Attorney General, was hospitalized with a severe abdominal illness. The condition, gallstone pancreatitis, is fairly common. Most patients do very well after this illness and completely recover. There are about 80,000 cases diagnosed annually in the United States and about 20 percent of the cases are severe.

WHAT IS PANCREATITIS? Pancreatitis is an inflammation of the pancreas. The pancreas is a gland that is located just behind the stomach and in the center of the abdomen, just below the breastbone. The function of the pancreas is to produce and secrete enzymes that help with the process of digestion. These enzymes help in the breakdown and digestion of fats, proteins, and carbohydrates in the small intestine. Also, the pancreas releases insulin into the bloodstream controlling blood sugar levels. A malfunctioning pancreas leads to the development of diabetes, but this is a separate and unrelated condition.

The digestive enzymes within the pancreas become active when they are secreted into the small intestine. During an episode of pancreatitis, the enzymes start working while they are contained within the gland and begin a process of "autodigestion." This is where the enzymes actually begin to digest and inflame the pancreas itself. This leads to severe pain and breakdown of the gland tissue.

WHAT ARE THE SYMPTOMS? The symptoms of pancreatitis include a sudden onset of pain in the area of the pancreas, just below the breastbone. The pain may come on after a large meal or excessive alcohol intake. The pain is constant, very sharp and may radiate into the back. Movement seems to worsen the pain and one may feel better by leaning forward. Additionally, there may be a fever, nausea, bloating, vomiting and a sense of restlessness.

HOW IS IT DIAGNOSED? The signs, symptoms, history and physical examination will usually give a clue to the health care provider that is evaluating the condition. Blood tests will be ordered to check for presence of infection. There are two specific enzyme levels of amylase and lipase, that will be tested. Elevation of one or both of these levels will help confirm the diagnosis. Finally, an ultrasound or CT scan of the abdomen will be completed. The results will show an enlarged, swollen and inflamed pancreas.

GASTRO-INTESTINAL

WHAT ARE THE CAUSES? Alcohol is the number one irritating factor for the development of pancreatitis. In the case of the Attorney General, a blockage in the pancreas caused by a gallstone prevented the release of the digestive enzymes. This is the second most common cause for pancreatitis. Other causes include medications, high cholesterol, trauma and cystic fibrosis.

WHAT IS THE TREATMENT? Once the diagnosis is made, the gastrointestinal tract must be rested. A patient may not be allowed to eat or drink anything for several days. A patient will be hydrated with intravenous fluids. Pain is the most bothersome symptom, so pain shots or intravenous pain medicines are given. In the presence of an infected gallbladder, intravenous antibiotics must be given.

Once the pancreas begins to cool down, surgery may be necessary to remove the gall bladder or gallstones that are causing the problem. A less invasive procedure may be performed using a fiber optic scope, where the blocked stone is identified and removed. The scope is inserted through the mouth and passed down through the stomach to identify the blockage.

Surgical intervention involving the pancreas itself should be avoided at all costs, because the pancreas is very sensitive to trauma. With pancreatitis, a patient may be hospitalized for a few days in order to get the condition under control. If alcohol is the irritating factor, life-long abstinence is usually necessary as one alcoholic drink may precipitate another case of pancreatitis.

WHAT ELSE SHOULD I DO? It is really important to follow the instructions that are given by your health care provider. Avoid alcohol and medications that may cause pancreatitis. If you have gallbladder disease and stones, surgical removal of the gall bladder may be necessary in order to prevent any further complications.

Pancreatitis is a very serious and life-threatening disease, but it usually has a good outcome if treatment is begun early in the process. Some changes in lifestyle may be necessary in order to prevent reoccurrence.

stomach flu
(a.k.a. gastroenteritis)

DR. WOJO'S PRESCRIPTION INSCRIPTION:
An explosion in your stomach is what you feel,
Rehydration is needed for you to heal.
Wash your hands and take it easy,
This should help you from feeling queasy.

Media coverage of "stomach flu" typically ranges from incidents on cruise ships, to school and community epidemics. There are a lot of myths about the stomach flu that I will attempt clear up.

WHAT IS STOMACH FLU? Stomach flu is actually a virus that infects the stomach and small intestine that typically lasts from one to three days. The word flu means influenza, so the terminology of stomach flu is actually a misnomer. Influenza is a specific respiratory illness not related to the gastrointestinal tract. The proper medical term is gastroenteritis.

WHAT ARE THE SYMPTOMS? Gastroenteritis can present with a variety of symptoms, but most commonly, patients experience nausea, stomach cramping, diarrhea, fever, chills and generalized aches and pains. In a mild case a person will only have a couple of the symptoms, but in a more severe case all of the symptoms may be present. Diarrhea is defined as two to four loose stools per day in an adult.

WHAT ARE THE CAUSES? Gastroenteritis can be caused by exposure to the infectious virus. This can occur through personal contact after which the virus is eventually swallowed. The exposure can also occur from secondary contact such as sharing utensils and food. This is the most common means of catching gastroenteritis.

Some of the common viruses that have been identified include adenovirus, rotavirus and the Norwalk virus. It is interesting to note that in over half of the cases that are medically evaluated, no specific cause is ever identified.

Other causes of gastroenteritis can include bacteria from food poisoning. It is also interesting to note that many people develop symptoms of the stomach flu after taking a course of antibiotics. Antibiotics can change the normal bacteria environment in the intestine. An imbalance of the different bacteria can lead to competition and overgrowth of a particular species. This eventually leads to symptoms of gastroenteritis. Some less common causes may be secondary to unusual bacteria, protozoa, handling of animals and reptiles, or chemical exposure.

GASTRO-INTESTINAL

HOW IS IT DIAGNOSED? Like so many medical conditions, gastroenteritis is a clinical diagnosis. It is especially easy for a health care provider to make the diagnosis in the face of a community epidemic. Depending on the facts surrounding the case, your provider may choose to complete some blood tests to rule out causes. A culture of the stool may be taken, but it may take three to five days to confirm a result. By this time, the condition has usually resolved itself! It is also important not to miss a more serious condition such as appendicitis, diverticulitis (intestinal wall inflammation and infection) or colitis.

WHAT HAPPENS? Once a virus or bacteria invade the stomach and intestines, the lining of these organs becomes inflamed. This irritation can cause spasm and inability to absorb foods and fluids. The intestines become hyperactive, moving food and water very quickly through the intestinal tract leading to diarrhea.

HOW IS IT TREATED? Once the diagnosis is made, the most important step is to rehydrate one's self. In more serious cases, an IV of salt water (saline) will be administered in the emergency department. The use of antinausea medicines may be given orally, intravenously or by rectal suppository. Most patients are sent home with an antinausea prescription and specific home instructions on diet.

Clear liquids are the mainstay of home treatment. Clear liquids are those that you can see through. Avoid dairy products, as these may prolong your condition. Other excellent home remedies include Gatorade and sport drinks. Once these liquids are well tolerated, the progression to a bland diet can occur. In children, the BRAT diet (bananas, rice, applesauce and toast) is a great starter.

In the event that a stool culture is positive for bacteria, your health care provider may need to prescribe an antibiotic in order to control the disease process. Fortunately, a large portion of these conditions is self-limited and will get better on their own.

WHAT SHOULD I DO? In the event that you experience gastroenteritis, you need to have a proper diagnosis made, especially to rule out other more serious illnesses. In the event that you have been exposed to "the stomach flu" in your community, you may choose to follow the above recommendations for rehydration and a bland diet. Resting the gastrointestinal tract is essential.

It is very important that you seek medical attention when faced with severe abdominal pain, dehydration, high fever, blood in the stools or generalized weakness. Also, do not forget to help prevent the spread of the illness with good hand washing and limiting close personal contact.

achilles tendon

One day, I played golf with a good friend and neighbor. I was surprised to see this athletic, fit young man ride in a golf cart and hobble up to the first tee. After he teed off and painfully made his way back to the golf cart, he told me that he had injured his Achilles tendon while on a long run at his cottage in the prior week.

My friend exercises, but apparently he outdid himself. He is now suffering from Achilles tendonitis, a fairly common problem that I often see as a physician.

WHAT IS ACHILLES TENDONITIS? This is a very painful and often debilitating irritation and inflammation of the heel cord. This tendon is the very large cord that goes over the back of the heel into the leg. The tendon attaches the calf muscles to the heel. These muscles allow for movement of the ankle. Without the use of this tendon, walking and running is nearly impossible.

When the Achilles tendon is injured, it is very painful and can be felt with every step. This may lead to swelling, weakness and inability to participate in simple standing, walking and running activities.

WHAT ARE THE SYMPTOMS? Achilles tendonitis comes on after excessive physical activity. The patient may complain of pain immediately after an activity or it may be present the next day. The pain and irritation will be located around the back of the heel, and there may be swelling. The pain may be sharp or dull and may extend into the back of the leg. Later signs of a more chronic problem may reveal the development of a lump in the area caused by the chronic inflammation.

WHAT CAUSES ACHILLES TENDONITIS? As was the case with my friend, excessive physical activity is the leading cause for this problem. Athletes are most commonly affected, followed by injured workers. The condition may develop after a single event or repetitive trauma. For example, walking or running on an uneven surface may lead to its development. Basketball and football players may experience this after sudden starts and stops. For the weekend warrior, improper and old shoe gear may be a factor.

INJURIES

Recent research has shown an association of Achilles tendonitis and the use of flouroquinolone antibiotics. These antibiotics have become commonplace in the treatment of a variety of infections.

HOW IS THIS DIAGNOSED? Your health care provider will assess your history of the pain and injury. Physical examination will be consistent with a painful Achilles tendon. Initially, x-rays are not taken unless severe trauma has occurred. In cases of prolonged and chronic problems, an MRI may be ordered to rule out any other more serious problems and confirm the diagnosis.

HOW IS THIS TREATED? Once the diagnosis is made, standard orthopedic treatment will be recommended. This includes avoiding irritating activities until the problem is completely resolved. Ice and the use of anti-inflammatory medications such as ibuprofen will be recommended. Many times, a ¼" heel lift will be prescribed to reduce the strain on the tendon. Usually, these simple measures will be enough to resolve the condition in a few weeks.

In chronic cases, more aggressive treatment will be recommended. This may involve a change of shoe gear, the use of custom-made foot orthotics, and physical therapy. Your health care provider may even choose one or two injections of a corticosteroid. Injections must be limited, as they may weaken the tendon.

The most severe cases may require complete rest of the tendon through the use of a cast for several weeks. Surgical correction to clean up the tendon is the last resort. Rehabilitation may take three months.

Overall, this is a fairly common and preventable problem. Gradually ease yourself into physical activities, but if you have the condition, be sure that you do not rush through the treatment as this nagging pain may bother you for a long period of time!

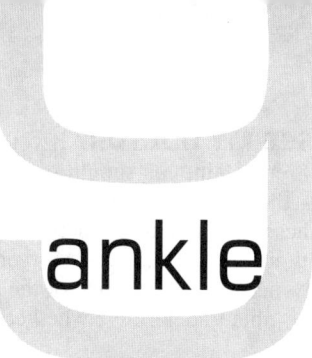

ankle

Ankle sprains are one of the most common injuries affecting both children and adults, in addition to being the most common musculoskeletal injury. In fact, sprains account for 25 percent of injuries seen in young athletes.

With the rising number of organized sports for youth such as baseball, football and soccer, the number of ankle sprains continues to grow. Even individual sporting activities, such as running, roller blading, scootering and snowboarding, contribute to these injuries.

WHAT IS AN ANKLE SPRAIN? To best understand what an ankle sprain actually is, let's talk about the parts that make up the ankle joint. The ankle is made up of three bones — the tibia (the inside ankle bone), the fibula (the outside ankle bone) and the talus (a hinge-type bone on top of the foot). Ligaments hold all of these bones together, making the joint stable. Ligaments can be stretched or torn, which makes the joint unstable and leaves it without support. A sprain is an injury to the joint exclusively involving the ligaments.

Ankle sprains can involve the inside of the ankle, the outside of the ankle, or both. By far the most common type of ankle sprain involves the outside of the ankle, which is caused when the foot and ankle twist inward and stretch the outside ligaments beyond their normal length.

WHAT IS THE TREATMENT? Emergency treatment for ankle sprains has been standard for years. The principle of RICE is applied — R is for Rest, I is for Ice, C is for Compression and E is for Elevation.

Resting the ankle is essential. Remember, "If it hurts, don't do it!" Next, apply ice to the injury. A good rule of thumb is 20 minutes on and 20 minutes off. Compression may involve a simple ACE bandage or an ankle support — both available at your local pharmacy. This moves any fluid out of the joint. Finally, it's important to elevate the injured ankle and avoid standing for long periods of time, because gravity will increase swelling. All of these steps should be followed immediately after injury, as well as during the healing phase. In general, it's best not to apply heat to a joint! This will increase pain and swelling in the injured ankle.

WHEN SHOULD I SEE MY DOCTOR? If you are unable to put weight on the ankle or are in extreme pain, you should see your doctor. In the ER, there are certain rules — the Ottawa Rules — that help the doctor determine if an x-ray is necessary. These rules evaluate whether the patient is able to walk more than four steps without assistance, and/or if there is pain in the tip of the anklebones and lastly, accounts for the age of the patient. Based on these observations, the doctor is able to determine whether there may be a fracture and if an x-ray is needed.

In the event that the injury is only a sprain, the doctor may recommend the use of an ACE wrap or an ankle support. Sometimes, crutches are recommended for more severe sprains. However, using crutches requires thorough instruction, and many people injure themselves while learning to use crutches, so I personally don't prescribe them unless absolutely necessary.

With more severe sprains, rehabilitation is important. Physical therapists are very skilled at returning patients to their pre-injury activity level. Very severe or recurrent ankle sprains may need surgery. During this procedure, an orthopedic surgeon uses tendons to reconstruct the joint. Typically this type of treatment is reserved for chronic ankle problems.

WHAT CAN I DO? When recuperating at home from a sprain, continue following the RICE therapy. Acetaminophen and ibuprofen are usually all that's needed for pain relief.

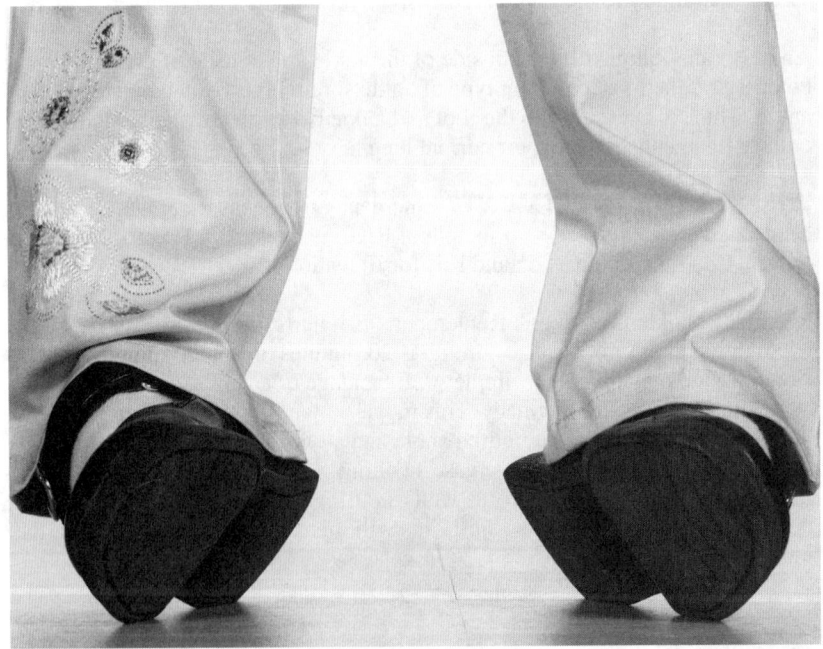

anterior
cruciate
ligament
(ACL)

According to post-operative reports, Carson Palmer, a Cincinnati Bengals quarterback sustained injuries to the internal and external ligaments of the knee, as well as dislocating his kneecap. A common injury that occurs with professional, collegiate, high school, and weekend warrior athletes is a rupture of the anterior cruciate ligament, referred to as the ACL.

WHAT IS THE ACL? This ligament is located inside the knee and it holds the femur, or thighbone, to the tibia, which is the weight-bearing shinbone of the lower leg. This ligament helps control movement of the knee and gives stability to the joint.

HOW DOES AN ACL INJURY OCCUR? Sporting activities such as football, soccer, basketball and skiing are the primary causes of injury. The knee may be forced in an abnormal direction when a fall results. Excessive twisting may occur, leading to damage. As with Palmer, his foot was planted on the turf of the football field and a 300-plus-pound lineman fell onto his leg. The force leads to stretching the knee beyond normal limits, resulting in a tear.

HOW IS THIS DIAGNOSED? A medical professional will assess the mechanism of injury and complete an examination. The patient will usually have a painful and swollen knee. A "pop" may have been felt at the time of the injury. The patient may feel unstable and have difficulty walking. The knee may feel like it wants to "go out of joint." After the exam, some x-rays may be in order. Plain x-rays are of no value in diagnosing an ACL tear. But they are helpful in find an associated fracture. The next most important x-ray is an MRI that can assess internal damage.

WHAT IS THE TREATMENT? Once the diagnosis is made, an evaluation by an orthopedic surgeon is in order. The orthopedist will outline treatment options based on the magnitude of the injury and lifestyle of the patient.

Conservative management and treatment may be recommended for a person with a rather sedentary lifestyle or minor injury. This will include physical therapy and strength training. Motivation of the patient is important. Also, a brace may be necessary when participating in some physical activities. The benefits of this recommendation are the avoidance of surgery, shorter recovery and usually the option to have surgical correction at a later date if necessary.

INJURIES

Active individuals with a severe injury will usually opt for surgical correction of the torn ligament. Statistics have shown over 90 percent success with surgery. The reconstruction may involve repair of the torn ligament directly or through use of a ligament graft. This will depend on many factors determined by your orthopedist.

Many of these surgical procedures can be completed through arthroscopy or scope, but your doctor will also determine this. After the surgery, physical therapy and rehabilitation are essential. The patient must be very motivated to participate in these activities, as well as very compliant. Usually, six to nine months of rehabilitation will be necessary until full recovery is achieved.

WHAT ELSE SHOULD BE DONE? If you sustain this injury, prompt medical attention is important. Initial treatment will involve ice, rest, a brace and pain medication. Then, visit an orthopedic surgeon that deals with this problem. Most orthopedists deal with this injury, but there are those that specialize in reconstruction surgery. You will be directed to the appropriate specialist after your initial evaluation.

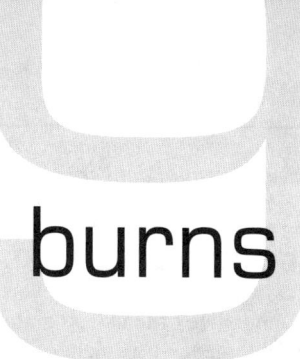

burns

Each year over one million people suffer thermal burns (burns caused by heat) in the U.S. About 75,000 of these patients are hospitalized, and 5,500 die as a result of these burns.

During the summer months, the number of burn cases grows due to outdoor activities such as camping, bonfires and the use of fireworks.

Children are the largest group afflicted with burns — over one-third of hospitalized burn patients are children! In fact, burns are the second leading cause of death for children between the ages of one and four.

WHAT ARE THE DIFFERENT TYPES OF BURNS, AND WHAT DO THEY LOOK LIKE? Burns are classified as first-, second-, and third-degree.

First-degree burns only involve the outer layer of the skin called the epidermis. These burns can be caused by the sun, scalds or fire flare-ups. The skin is red, dry and painful. When treating a first-degree burn, it's best to cool the skin as quickly as possible and take medication, like acetaminophen or aspirin, as necessary to relieve the pain. In general, first-degree burns do not require professional medical attention. These burns will heal just fine on their own.

Second-degree burns involve the underlying skin called the dermis. These burns are caused by significant splash injuries, scalds, immersions or brief flame burns. They may appear pink, moist, include fluid-filled blisters and are extremely painful, but they will usually not scar. As with first-degree burns, cooling the skin quickly and taking medication to relieve the pain is your best course of action. Follow-up care involves cleaning the burn and applying antibiotic creams.

The most severe burns, third-degree burns, destroy both the epidermis and dermis. Third-degree burns can be caused by significant scalds, prolonged flame exposure and high voltage electrical exposure. The skin appears dry, white, charred and leather-like. Third-degree burns destroy the nerve endings, so they are not painful. Scarring occurs, so skin grafting, a procedure that removes skin from other parts of the body to cover the burned area, will be needed.

INJURIES

> *Since many burns are due to acts of carelessness, prevention truly is most important. Be sure to survey potential dangers around your home to decrease the chances of getting burned!*

WHAT SHOULD I DO ABOUT SEVERE BURNS? The first 24 hours of care are the most critical when dealing with severe third-degree burns. It is important to call 911. The police officers and ambulance personnel that respond are trained in the emergency treatment of burns. They make sure that the victim's airway remains open, fluids are replaced, the wound is properly treated, and the victim receives medication to relieve pain.

For severely-burned patients, emergency care will be continued at the hospital. Many emergency doctors have special training and certifications in burn treatment. Eventually, patients with extensive burns may need to be transferred to a specialized burn center, but the most critical portion of treatment takes place during this initial emergency care.

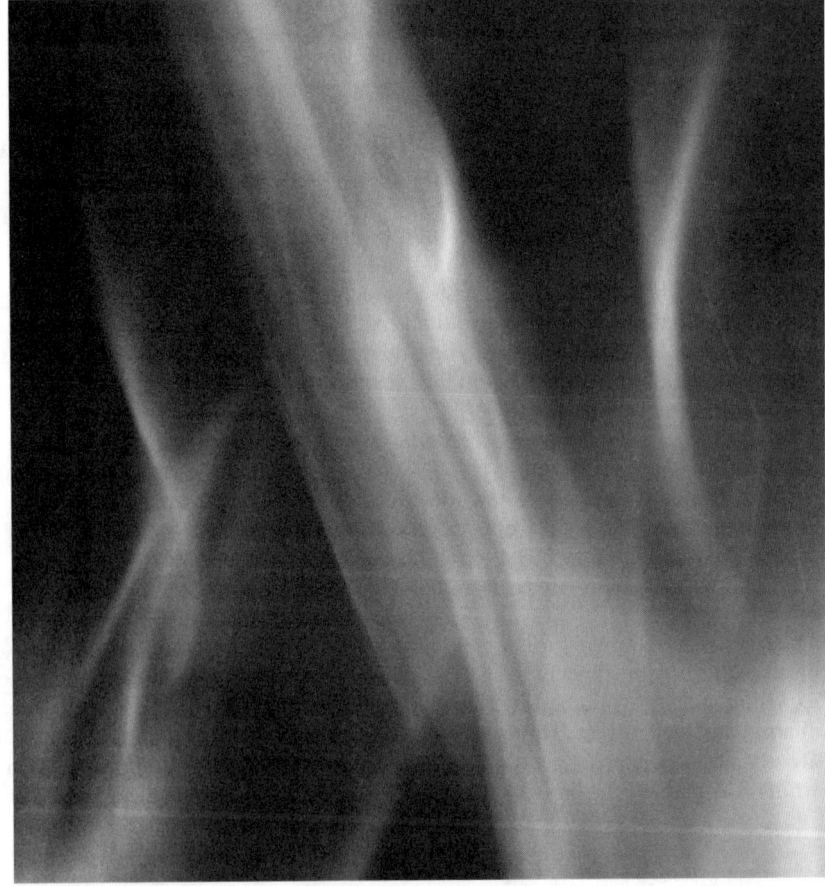

gardening

With the approach of spring, outdoor activities once again become the norm, including a variety of sporting activities and yard work. My wife is always excited to start on the yard, flower beds and vegetable garden and usually a few doses of ibuprofen! Gardening activities account for about 400,000 tool-related injuries each year.

WHAT ARE THE MOST COMMON INJURIES? The start of a new season can lead to a variety of injuries that may be due to deconditioning. Most commonly, over-zealous gardeners may present with a variety of back complaints and wrist complaints. The common backache is usually due to overuse and bending for a prolonged period of time. The practice of good body mechanics will prevent this. Be sure to take frequent breaks while in the garden and bent over. Do not lift more than you can handle and when you do lift, use your legs and not your back. Seek help when lifting heavy objects such as large potted plants.

Another common overuse injury involves the wrist, including tendonitis and carpal tunnel syndrome. When the wrist is exposed to repetitive twisting and turning over a prolonged period, the tendons surrounding the wrist may become inflamed. Be cognizant of these prolonged motions, as you may suffer for a couple of weeks with an inflamed wrist that will only get better with rest, ice and ibuprofen.

Mechanized gardening and yard tools may have an excessive amount of vibration. Prolonged use of these tools may lead to the development of carpal tunnel syndrome. Carpal tunnel involves trapping of a nerve that goes through the wrist into the hand. When this occurs, the thumb, index and long finger may become numb. This may require the use of a night splint or surgery. Be sure to use tools with big padded handles and do not overdo it when you are out in the yard.

Protect your hands when you are outside. Wear comfortable leather gloves. This will prevent your hands from being cut by branches or other objects in the soil. Diabetics are at even greater risk of breaking skin and getting an infection, so they should be very cautious and protect their hands. You will also be protected from insects, snakes or other rodents that may fight back when you invade their territory. Raccoons, skunks, bats, foxes and coyotes have the highest incidence of rabies, so stay clear of these animals. Usually squirrels, chipmunks, mice and rabbits are not infected.

In the north, many of us have not been exposed to the sun all winter, so a couple days outside can lead to sunburn. Protect your skin and wear 30+ SPF sunscreen. If you are burned, aspirin is still a great way to relieve yourself of the pain.

WHAT ARE THE SEVERE GARDENING INJURIES? Many garden and lawn tools are dangerous to operate, especially if you are inexperienced. It is essential to keep all safety guards on lawn mowers, rotor tillers, chain saws, weed whackers and chippers. These tools can lead to an amputation of a finger, toe or extremity. Use these tools as they have been designed and do not take shortcuts. Most of the injuries that I see are because the patient took a shortcut and improperly used a tool.

Protect your eyes and ears at all times. Eye injuries occur from debris flying out of a lawn mower or other garden tool. Also, most of these tools are very noisy and require the use of ear protection. Prolonged exposure to many of these noises can lead to permanent hearing loss.

Most of us cannot wait for the spring and summer months. Take the time to condition and protect yourself so that you can enjoy this time to the fullest.

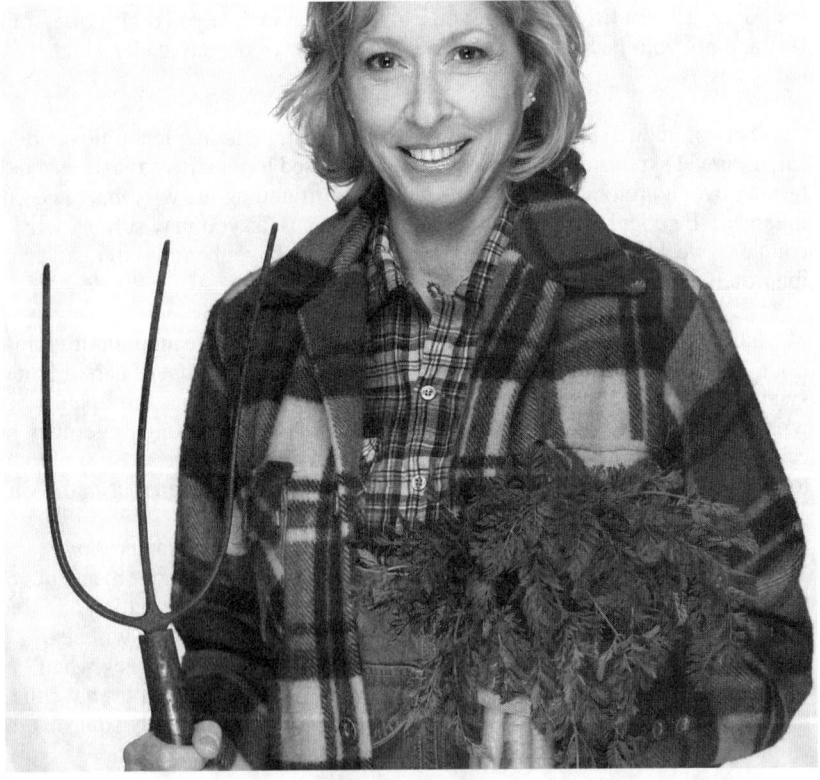

To Your Health with Dr. Wojo

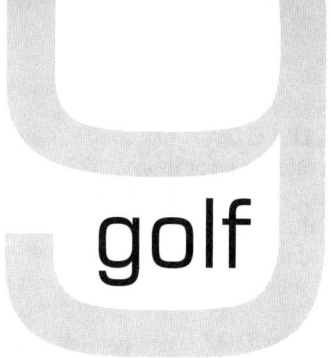

golf

Each year, as I attempt to improve my golf handicap (and never do!), I discover some muscles that I missed during my daily aerobic and weight lifting workout. Regardless, preparing for the golf season does require a great deal of time and effort. As a result, some golfers may sustain a variety of injuries.

There are over 40 million golfers worldwide, and over 80 percent will sustain some form of injury while playing this sport. It is hard to believe that a benign sport such as golf can contribute to a wide variety of injuries. While most are not serious, many can be chronic and end one's season prematurely.

WHAT ARE COMMON GOLF INJURIES? Over 80 percent of all golf injuries are related to overuse, while less than 20 percent are due to direct trauma. Most of the overuse use injuries are due to the stresses that are placed on the neck, back, shoulder, elbow and wrist. These types of injuries are quite similar among professional and amateur golfers.

Injuries due to direct trauma are less frequent, but a golf ball striking an individual is the most common injury. Being struck by a club during the swing follows this. These injuries are certainly much more serious and can leave a golfer with a life-long disability.

HOW CAN THIS BE PREVENTED? A study in the American Journal of Sports Medicine has shown that a 10-minute warm-up routine can decrease the chances of a chronic overuse injury.

It is very important to understand the biomechanics of golf and the first preventative measure is taking lessons. It is essential to learn to properly swing a club. A great deal of force is transferred through the neck, back, shoulders, elbows, wrists and legs during the swing. Improper body position can attribute to muscle and joint injury.

WHAT ELSE SHOULD I DO? It has been shown that golfers that rush to their tee time are at greater risk for injury. This may be initiated by yanking the heavy golf bag from the car and running off to the first tee. It has been shown that these golfers need at least four holes to settle down. So, take your time and prepare for the game, as you may spare yourself injury and even a few strokes!

HOW SHOULD I WARM UP? Spend at least 10 minutes walking, stretching, and swinging your clubs. Focus on all aspects of the body, from head to toe. A daily stretching routine improves flexibility and lessens the chance for injury.

Muscle strengthening is essential and many professionals have improved their game through weight training and improving overall muscle balance. For example, strengthening the shoulder has led to a decrease in rotator cuff injuries.

OVERUSE IS OVERUSE! Be careful that you don't spend too much time on the practice range and practice green. Adequate rest is essential and as with so many orthopedic conditions, "if it hurts, don't do it!"

For example, many people develop golfer's elbow through repeated irritation with the golf swing. Pain is noted in the elbow as the arm pulls the club through the swing or with repeated strikes to the ground. Be careful to avoid this pitfall.

WHAT ABOUT COMMON SENSE? So much of this information is common sense. With regard to direct trauma, the golfer must always be aware of other golfers and their swing path. Stay clear of your golfing buddies on the tee box.

Alcohol frequently plays a role in many of the injuries. Be sure to limit alcohol intake, as this does affect coordination. In addition, alcohol contributes to dehydration on hot summer days. Be very cautious in drinking alcohol on the course and be prepared for a safe trip home.

Lastly, in the event of bad weather, stay home! If a storm comes up while on the course, immediately head to the clubhouse or take shelter. Numerous lightning strikes occur on the golf course annually leading to permanent disability and death. Do not take any chances.

Golf is a wonderful sport for everyone. It is also a great family sport. Take time to learn the game, warm up appropriately and use common sense. This is not a handicap!

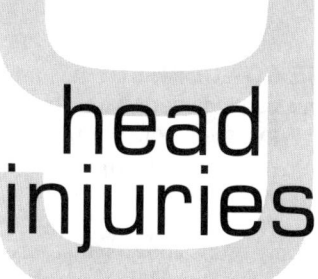

head injuries

Each year, over a half million children are seen in our nation's emergency departments for head injuries and about 20 percent of these patients are admitted to the hospital. Unfortunately, about 7,000 children die annually from head trauma and almost 30,000 suffer permanent disabilities.

Fortunately, a great deal of children seen have minor trauma that results in no long-term consequences. The most common injury sustained is a concussion. As friends or family members, our goal is to protect children from unnecessary injuries. However, when accidents happen, physicians do their best to prevent permanent complications.

WHAT IS A CONCUSSION? A concussion is a type of brain injury that involves a change in mental status with or without loss of consciousness. There can be a variety of symptoms that accompany this injury including headache, dizziness, confusion or amnesia. Many times, this term is used as a general description for a variety of head injuries.

WHAT HAPPENS? With very young children, the skull's soft spot does not immediately close in the head, which allows the skull to expand and helps the child to withstand greater injury with less chance of severe head injury. Many times a very young child can withstand greater injury than adults. However, children under one who suffer a head trauma have a higher death rate because of delayed treatment. It is difficult to diagnose a severe brain injury due to the child's inability to communicate their pain and concerns.

Compared to adults, children have a lower incidence of bleeding in the brain and swelling. Their injuries are usually due to shearing force that causes bruising. This puts the child at increased risk for seizures after the accident. The seizures can occur only during the period of injury, but can potentially be long lasting.

INJURIES

WHEN SHOULD I BE CONCERNED? It is important to assess how the injury occurred. A fall on a carpeted floor with a bruise to the forehead is not as significant as a fall on a concrete floor. Sporting injuries are also frequently a source of concussions. Symptoms to watch for include the loss of consciousness, confusion, irritability, headache, nausea, vomiting and sleepiness.

If the injury is severe and any of the above symptoms appear, it is important that you seek medical advice for your child. Your doctor will need to evaluate the injury and determine the right course of treatment, which may include x-rays.

WHAT SHOULD I EXPECT? If the injury is serious, the goal of your doctor is to prevent the injury from getting worse. However, many times it is difficult to determine how serious the head injury is.

It is important that every child receives individualized treatment. If an x-ray is needed, a CT scan must be completed. A CT scan is a rapid x-ray scanner able to look at the brain internally, as well as the skull.

The CT scan will show if there is bleeding, bruising or a fracture. The physician is then able to decide on the appropriate action. Of course, all children do not need to be scanned. A child that has not had symptoms after a head injury can be safely observed.

WHAT ARE SOME POSSIBLE TREATMENTS? If there is bleeding or swelling in the brain, surgery may be needed to stop the bleeding and relieve swelling. IV medications may also be used to reduce swelling. Many times an internal monitor will be placed in the brain to monitor pressure.

With minor injuries, observation is the key to treatment. This may involve an overnight stay at the hospital or close observation at home. Appropriate management of pain can be accomplished with the use of Tylenol.

WHAT CAN I DO? Like with so many childhood emergencies, prevention is essential. It is important that children be trained to wear appropriate headgear such as bicycle helmets. They must be restrained in the car at all times. In addition, appropriate education of children will make them sensitive to these issues.

Head injuries have a wide range of consequences. They can be prevented, but if your child is faced with this unfortunate injury, please seek medical attention. The results can mean a difference for a lifetime!

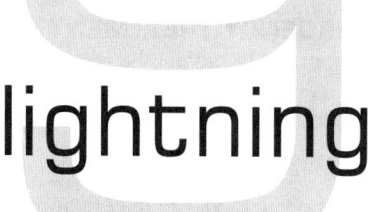

lightning

Lightning, a very dangerous natural hazard, is also a dangerous health hazard that must be taken seriously. Injuries caused by a lightning strike may occur in a matter of seconds and without warning. These strikes can also easily contribute to permanent disability or death. Thus, when the threat of a thunderstorm is eminent, cover should be sought immediately.

HOW COMMON ARE THUNDERSTORMS? During every minute of every day, there are at least 1,800 thunderstorms occurring somewhere in the world. In the United States, about 400 people are struck each year and nearly 100 people die after being struck by lightning. In addition to this, several people will suffer a long-term disability after the strike.

During the summer months, thunderstorms are very common. Lightning can strike 10 miles away from a rainstorm. It is important to remember that if thunder is heard, there is lightning. It is really important to watch for dark clouds and increasing wind. This may be an indication of an impending storm.

HOW STRONG IS LIGHTNING? The magnitude of lightning is tremendous. The streak of the electrical current can extend up to five miles. The temperature of a strong strike can reach a temperature of 50,000° F. The average lightning strike is about 30,000 amperes, but the electricity flowing in a bolt can reach up to 200 million volts.

WHO GETS INJURED? Being outside is the greatest risk for injury from lightning. In the United States, one third of the victims are injured while at work, one third are injured during recreational and athletic activities, and the last third are injured in a variety of situations.

WHAT ARE THE INJURIES? Lightning injuries are electrical injuries. The heart and the brain are the most common organs affected. A strike can contribute to a cardiac arrhythmia, or irregular beating of the heart. Left untreated, this will lead to death.

Electrical injuries burn the body. Muscles can be damaged, as well as nerves. The electrical strike can also affect the brain causing altered memory, difficulty concentrating, irritability and even a personality change.

WHAT IS THE EMERGENCY TREATMENT? As with most emergency situations, it is important to protect the rescuer prior to tending to the victim, as additional injury should be avoided. It is essential to call 911. Help will be on the way. Emergency workers are well trained in dealing with this type of situation.

Since cardiac arrhythmias occur, a victim may require CPR until additional medical assistance arrives. Then, more definitive medical treatment will be provided probably including a visit to the emergency department. If a patient has been burned, fluids will be provided intravenously and a transfer to a burn center may be in order. A comprehensive medical evaluation must be completed to assess all of the injuries.

HOW DO I PREVENT LIGHTNING INJURIES? Several safety rules are recommended during a thunderstorm. Go inside immediately! Be sure that you are in a low point, as lightning strikes the highest point of an area.

Do not wait for rain to start before seeking shelter. If there is thunder, there is lightning. It is very important during athletic activities to suspend the practice or game IMMEDIATELY if thunder is heard. The risk of lightning strike is very high. Stay away from trees.

If water sports are involved, get out of and away from water. Get out of a metal boat and off the water as soon as possible. People on the water are prime targets. In addition, lightning strikes can travel through plumbing, so avoid showers, baths and laundry during a storm.

Most importantly, stay informed about the path of a storm through local radio and television broadcasts, as well as NOAA Weather Radio. Prevention is the best medicine when dealing with this deadly weather phenomenon!

To Your Health with Dr. Wojo

sports hernia

Donovan McNabb, of the Philadelphia Eagles, was sidelined because of a sports hernia, a fairly common injury in male athletes.

WHAT IS A SPORTS HERNIA? Just like any hernia, a sports hernia involves the weakening or tearing of a muscle. The sports hernia is located in the groin, just above the inguinal ligament. The inguinal ligament is located in the crease of the hip and the leg. The injury involves a tearing of the abdominal wall just above the inguinal ligament, leading to pain in this area. This is similar to another common type of hernia known as the inguinal hernia. But, unlike the inguinal hernia, a sports hernia usually does not involve a big bulge.

WHAT CAUSES THIS? Over the years, sports hernias have been more frequently diagnosed in high school, collegiate and professional athletes. Sporting activities that involve a great deal of twisting and turning at high speeds usually are the culprit. The most common sports that lead to these hernias are soccer, hockey and football.

Studies have shown that men are much more frequently affected than women. It is unclear if this is because the offending sporting activities are more male dominated or if there is truly an anatomical difference that may protect women from this type of injury.

WHAT ARE THE SYMPTOMS? A sports hernia may be difficult to diagnose. Initially, an athlete may complain of deep groin pain and there may be no coinciding physical findings. The pain will be on one side and may be initially noticed while getting in and out of a car. Usually, the pain begins during physical activity and may last during exercise. It may go away when the activity has ceased.

As the condition worsens and progresses, pain may be noted throughout the day and night and associated with activities of daily living. It is interesting to note that in many of the cases, the onset is insidious. But there are some athletes that are able to pinpoint the exact injury, which involves a tearing sensation in the lower abdominal wall. Thus, there may be abdominal wall tenderness with radiation of the pain into the testicles in males.

INJURIES

HOW IS IT DIAGNOSED? In recent years, health professionals have become more aware of the sports hernia. The onset of pain without physical findings in an athlete should lead a health care provider to pursue this diagnosis. As always, the historical perspective of the injury and symptoms are essential.

Physical examination of an athlete with a sports hernia may reveal no obvious deformity. But the clinician must rule out other medical problems that may be causing groin pain. This may involve a muscle strain, other hernias, chip fracture, bursitis or tendonitis.

Usually, diagnostic testing such as x-rays are of little value to find a sports hernia, but they are helpful in ruling out other problems. A CT scan or an MRI will assess internal structures and may show the sports hernia. Most importantly, the examiner must take all of the patient information and clinically correlate it to make the diagnosis.

WHAT IS THE TREATMENT? Research has shown that rest and rehabilitation may help the condition. Strengthening exercises and physical therapy may improve the symptoms. This is a long process that halts the participation of the athlete.

The most definitive treatment is surgery. With the advent of laparoscopic surgery, the procedure is very safe and quite simple. Many times, this surgical intervention is diagnostic, as the diagnosis is not very clear-cut.

The post-operative period must involve 6 to 12 weeks of rehabilitation and strengthening. An athlete may return to full participation in this time frame. Recovery is usually complete with no problems.

Prevention is essential and athletes at risk must train appropriately. This involves strength training of the lower abdomen, pelvis and hips. A guided workout by a trained professional is important. Medical attention is important if you are concerned that you may have this problem.

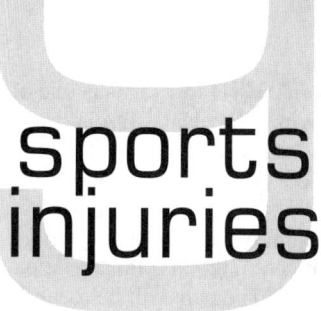

sports injuries

For some students, summer is restful and without a lot of organized physical activity. Thus, appropriate preparation and conditioning will be necessary for the fall sporting activities. A couple of common overuse injuries that we see early on in the season are shin splints and plantar fasciitis. These are injuries of the lower extremities.

WHAT ARE SHIN SPLINTS? This is a generalized term that refers to pain on the front of the leg. This is not a specific diagnosis, but a description of symptoms. The most common area of pain is over the tibia or shinbone. This is the firm surface of the inside portion of the lower leg. What usually occurs is that the lining of the bone, called the periostium, becomes elevated off the bone and inflamed. Usually, the traction forces of the muscles in the leg will irritate this area due to overuse.

Shin splints may also be due to a stress fracture of the lower leg, which could be a tiny crack in the bone. When the outer portion of the lower leg becomes inflamed, this is referred to as lateral shin splints. This is caused by a muscular strain.

With shin splints, a person may develop lower leg pain after excessive activity, especially in unconditioned participants. There may be some swelling over the lower leg with some associated redness. These symptoms may come on after excessive running, overtraining, running uphill or jumping. The muscle groups of the lower extremity are simply overworked.

When this happens, rest is essential. Additional treatment may include physical therapy, stretching, massage, icing and stretching. A trip to the doctor may involve a comprehensive assessment of the cause of the problem. Many people have excessive pronation of the foot, which is an abnormal rolling of the foot inward. This abnormal motion translates into problems in the lower leg. Thus, your health care provider may prescribe custom arch supports and an anti-inflammatory such as ibuprofen.

WHAT IS PLANTAR FASCIITIS? This is one of the most common causes of heel and arch pain. The plantar fascia is a long band of tissue that starts at the underside of the heel and extends to the ball of the foot. This tissue gives support to the foot and becomes inflamed with over-activity.

The most common complaint is that the patient will note severe pain in the heel when hopping out of bed in the morning. The pain will usually subside a little with increased activity. The pain will be localized to the heel or the arch.

It is not completely understood what causes plantar fasciitis. Overuse may contribute to the problem, as well as trauma. There may be some biomechanical abnormalities in the foot leading to excessive stretching of the plantar fascia.

This can be a difficult problem to treat and symptoms may persist for six months or more. Usually, rest, ice and limiting the abnormal forces on the foot will cure the problem. A trip to the local podiatrist or orthopedic surgeon with more severe cases may involve a prescription of custom arch supports called orthotics. Sometimes an injection of an anti-inflammatory steroid will help. Additionally, physical therapy may shorten the recovery period. It is most important that the foot be rested until completely recovered. Surgery is seldom indicated and has limited success in a few cases.

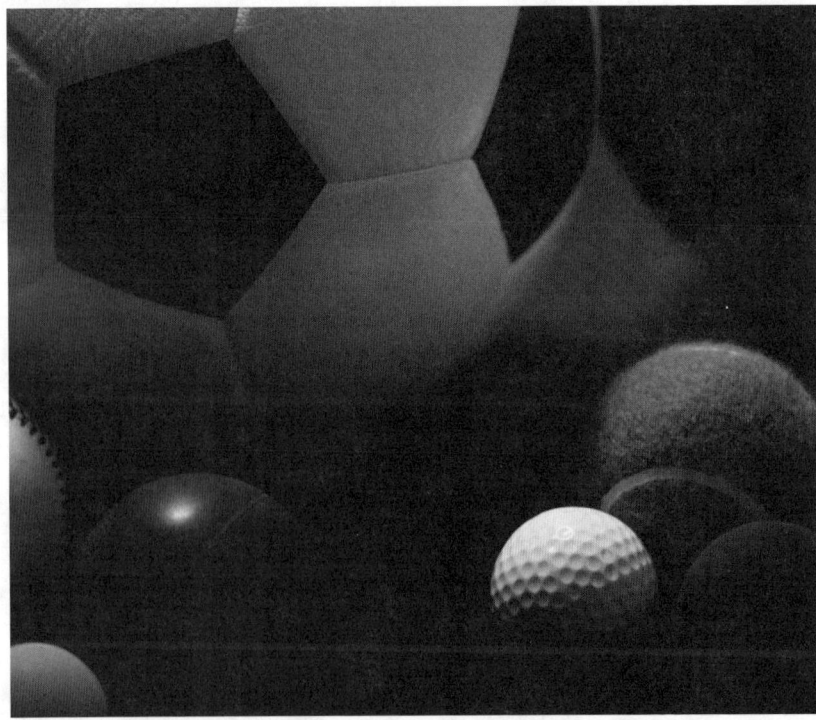

water intoxication

Recently, a woman and mother of three died senselessly in California due to water intoxication. She actually drank herself to death while participating in a radio station contest to see who could drink the most water without going to the bathroom. She took second in the contest and was found dead a little later in the day, after stating that she had a bad headache.

The woman died from water intoxication. This is a medical entity that is well known and the radio station was warned of this complication.

WHAT IS WATER INTOXICATION? This is a condition, known as hyperhydration, whereby a person takes in a large volume of water in a very short period of time. The electrolytes of the body—most specifically sodium—are diluted. This causes a shift in the concentration of the body's chemicals and water is sucked into the body's cells. The rapid intake of the water into the cells will cause them to explode. This leads to grave consequences because body organs are damaged.

If a person is on a normal diet and consumes about three quarts of water at a single sitting, they will develop water intoxication. If the individual maintains a low sodium diet, about a quart and a half of water can prove fatal.

WHAT ARE THE SYMPTOMS? As was the case in California, a person who has taken in too much water will experience light-headedness, weakness, abdominal pain nausea, and vomiting. Eventually, the most serious consequence will be a sudden onset of brain swelling with an associated headache. Then a person will have seizures and go into a coma. Death is the final step. The entire process will occur in a few short hours, as the water is rapidly absorbed from the intestines into the blood stream.

WHO IS AT RISK? Any individual who consumes a large volume of water during a very short period of time is at risk. Throughout the years, several people have died after participating in stunts such as the one in California. Coed students have died after being involved in hazing and initiation rituals for fraternities.

However, a variety of other people are at risk as well. Several studies have looked at marathon runners who have died during a race or shortly thereafter. During a long hot race, runners will lose sodium and drink only water. The sodium levels rapidly diminish due to sweating and then are further diluted by drinking only water that does not replenish electrolytes. When a runner collapses, it is often thought that they have suffered a heart attack, but this may not be the case. Similar circumstances can surround an individual who is working in a hot environment and only drinking water.

Patients with psychiatric illness are also at risk. Some of the psychiatric medications taken can lead to an increased water intake. Other medical problems that may lead to water intoxication are secondary to kidney disease. It has also been shown that drug abusers will drink large volumes of water in order to taint an upcoming drug test. Many times, they do not survive to complete the test.

WHAT IS THE TREATMENT? When a known case is diagnosed, the initial treatment involves replacing sodium with intravenous, normal saline. Next, a diuretic will be given to rid the body of water. A diuretic is a water excreting medication. More severe cases can be given other medications that are used to balance out the electrolytes and water.

Ultimately, prevention is the most important step in avoiding water intoxication. Avoid stunts that promote drinking large quantities of water in a short period of time. The radio staff in California was warned about the dangers of water intoxication and they were all fired. They are also facing criminal charges of homicide, despite thinking that they would be immune since the contestant signed a release.

Athletes should not solely drink water to quench their thirst. They should drink appropriate fluids, such as sports drinks, that are well balanced with electrolytes. Workers in hot environments should follow the same practices.

If one is concerned that they may be experiencing water intoxication, medical attention should be sought immediately. This is truly an emergency.

To Your Health with Dr. Wojo

back pain

One of the most common reasons that a person with a musculoskeletal complaint will visit the doctor or the emergency room is for lower back pain. This is also one of the most common reasons that employees miss work.

WHAT CAUSES A BACKACHE? There are over 200 muscles that support the spinal column, which consists of several bones called vertebrae. Ligaments attach these vertebrae along with a pad that is found between each bone. All of these elements hold the human body in an upward posture. In addition, nerves exit from the spinal cord through these bones.

Back pain will result with overuse and strain of these muscles and ligaments. The stress on the muscles will not allow the body to be maintained in an upright posture and pain will persist. The nerves can become irritated leading to additional discomfort. With more severe cases, numbness and weakness of the extremities can occur.

In general, a backache may be caused by overuse of the muscles. This stretching and straining may lead to muscle spasm and pain. Usually, this type of pain is self-limited and will resolve with rest. Other conditions must be considered, such as arthritis, nerve damage, infection, kidney stones or tumor. Some of these conditions are less likely, but must always be considered.

WHAT ARE THE SYMPTOMS? Pain in the back may occur anywhere along the spinal column. This pain may range from a dull ache to a severe, sharp, stabbing feeling. There may be some radiation of pain into the buttocks and the legs. Pain will worsen with movement, coughing, sneezing or straining.

In the event that the symptoms progress to severe pain in the legs, knees or feet, a pinched nerve or herniated disk may be present. If there is accompanying weakness, loss of function of the legs, or loss of bowel and bladder control, immediate medical attention is required.

WHAT DIAGNOSTIC TESTING IS REQUIRED? With straightforward cases of back pain, no testing is required. Obtaining a good history and physical examination are the mainstay of the medical evaluation. Usually your health care provider will treat the symptoms and wait for improvement. In the event that the condition has not improved within a week or so, further testing may be required.

PAIN

Plain x-rays of the back are usually of little value. They will only show arthritic changes or changes from trauma. The most useful test is an MRI x-ray. This shows the bony and soft tissue structures such as the muscles, ligaments and disks– information that helps clarify the root of the problem.

WHAT CAN I DO? In the event that the back pain is caused by overuse, simple home remedies such as rest, heat, nonsteroidal anti-inflammatory medications like ibuprofen and the use of Tylenol will help resolve the condition. It may take a week or two to be completely asymptomatic.

In the event that the simple home remedies are not successful, a visit to your health care provider may be necessary. A review of your medical history and a physical examination will help your medical professional make an appropriate diagnosis. Prescription medications of nonsteroidal anti-inflammatories and narcotics may be indicated.

It may be helpful to undergo a course of physical therapy. Different treatments may be provided, as well as stretching exercises and home exercises. With more serious cases, an evaluation by a back specialist may be necessary. With severe pain caused by a slipped or herniated disk, surgery may be necessary to correct the problem.

CAN BACK PAIN BE PREVENTED? Yes. It is important to exercise and maintain good physical conditioning. Appropriate techniques for lifting and not over-exerting one's self are essential. With recurrent back problems, your health care provider and physical therapist can prescribe back strengthening exercises. In the event that your condition worsens and is not responding to the above conservative efforts, a visit to your health care provider is in order.

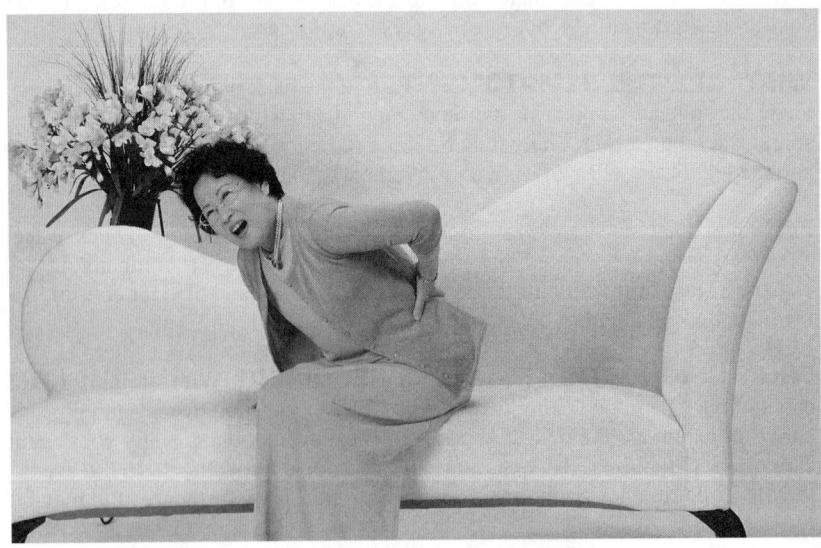

complex regional pain syndrome (CRPS)

It was reported that Paula Abdul suffered from an eating disorder and chronic pain syndrome. More specifically, it was noted that she has suffered from Complex Regional Pain Syndrome (CRPS), formerly know as Reflex Sympathetic Dystrophy or Causalgia.

WHAT IS CRPS? This is a fairly uncommon condition that usually affects an arm or leg, resulting in severe uncontrollable pain. Other body parts can be affected as well. This is a disorder of the peripheral nerves and the central nervous system.

When a body part is affected, there will be severe pain in the area, changes in the appearance of the skin, inability to move the body part and changes in temperature of the skin. These changes may occur slowly or rapidly after an injury, surgery or other vascular type of event.

WHAT CAUSES CRPS? The actual cause of this disease is unclear, but it is thought that the nerve responses in the reflex arc are interrupted. Untoward events that may contribute to its development may include an extremity sprain or fracture. It is interesting to note that up to 35 percent of all cases have no known exposure to a bad event.

About 20 percent of patients with CRPS may have experienced a heart attack or stroke. Medical procedures such as back or knee surgery may cause this as well. Type I cases are caused by a soft tissue injury and Type II cases are caused by a direct nerve injury.

WHO IS AFFECTED? Medical studies have shown that both men and women can be affected, but clearly more women than men are afflicted. The most common age group of patients are young women.

WHAT ARE THE SIGNS AND SYMPTOMS? After an injury, patients may complain of pain that is out of proportion to physical findings. This may be the first indication of CRPS. A patient may note very severe, burning pain. The skin may be very sensitive to the touch.

PAIN

Eventually, the skin may become shiny, cool and sweaty. As time progresses, hair will be lost from the affected extremity and there may be changes in the finger or toenails. The extremity may stiffen up and lose the ability to move. This may lead to muscle spasms, weakness and loss of muscle known as atrophy.

HOW IS THIS DIAGNOSED? The clinical history is very important, especially if there is a prior direct injury to the affected body part. Once a clinician has seen a case of CRPS, it is not difficult to miss. Confirmatory tests may include nerve studies, plain x-ray and bone scans. The x-ray tests reveal a very classic appearance in the change of the boney structure.

WHAT IS THE TREATMENT? As there is no cure for CRPS, preventing progression of the disease process is essential. Treatment is aimed at alleviating the severe pain that is associated with the problem and preventing symptoms from getting worse. Physical therapy is a very important treatment, especially in helping with the range of motion of the affected extremity.

Psychotherapy may be necessary to help a patient mentally deal with the pain. Sometimes, a nerve block will help in diminishing the pain. A wide variety of medications such as the nonsteroidal anti-inflammatory drugs, narcotics, antidepressants and antiseizure medications may help.

As a last resort, surgically cutting the affected nerves may help in controlling the pain. More recently, the use of spinal cord stimulators and drug pumps inserted into the spinal canal have shown promise.

HOW LONG WILL THIS LAST? Most cases will resolve in six to nine months, if caught early and treated aggressively. Unfortunately, some patients may experience a prolonged course if they do not seek early treatment. Some cases may relapse as well.

Thus, it is important to seek medical attention if you experience some of the unusual symptoms noted after experiencing trauma to a body part. To learn more about ongoing research and current treatment methods, go to www.rsds. org.

fentanyl

In 2005, the United States Food and Drug Administration (FDA) issued a warning to health care providers to caution them when prescribing the powerful painkiller, transdermal fentanyl. Since it became available in December 1990, there have been 120 recorded deaths, which have been thought to be secondary to overdosage. Deaths have occurred with both forms of the medication marketed as Duragesic and as the generic fentanyl.

WHAT IS FENTANYL? Fentanyl is a very strong pain reliever that is used primarily with chronic pain patients and is delivered in patch form. Most people are familiar with morphine and this is similar to it, but more potent. It comes in oral, injectable and transdermal forms. The transdermal formulation is the one that has received national attention.

Duragesic was originally sold and marketed by Janssen Pharmaceuticals, a division of Johnson and Johnson. In 2004, it was reported that there were over $2 billion in sales of this medication alone. In 2005, Mylan Laboratories began to sell the generic form. In 2005, Johnson and Johnson notified clinicians of the potential for misuse and abuse of this drug. Now the FDA is conducting an investigation into the deaths that have occurred.

WHAT ARE THE INDICATIONS FOR USE? Fentanyl is used to manage moderate and severe forms of pain. It is usually prescribed to patients with chronic pain problems or those with severe cancer pain. The use of the patch form allows for steady, consistent delivery of the medication over a three-day period. The patch must be removed after three days and then replaced.

WHAT ARE THE SAFETY ISSUES? With any narcotic pain reliever, over dosage can occur. Fentanyl should be initially prescribed in the lowest dosage and closely monitored. Also, this medication is not clinically indicated for short-term usage or for pain that is not constant.

It is important to remember that this medication should be used with people that have not been relieved by short-term oral pain medications. There is an addictive potential, so caution must be exercised.

PAIN

When using the patch, it must be used exactly as prescribed. Follow the directions that come with the package insert and those given by the doctor and pharmacist. Proper storage will prevent damage to the patch, that could alter the delivery mechanism. Be sure to protect children from getting this potentially dangerous medicine. Most importantly, too much of this medicine can lead to a life-threatening overdose.

WHAT ARE THE SIGNS OF OVERDOSE? As with any narcotic pain medication, too much medicine can depress breathing. One may see a slowed respiratory pattern, extreme sleepiness or tiredness, loss of clear thought process, or even respiratory arrest. Any symptoms indicate the need for immediate medical attention.

The levels of fentanyl can be elevated in one's body when combined with some medicines affecting brain function. It has been shown that when fentanyl builds up, it may take nearly a day to clear from the system. Also, the use of alcohol with fentanyl is strictly prohibited, as they may have a combined and unwanted effect.

Pain medicines have an effect on the gastrointestinal tract. This may lead to slowing of the bowel with obstruction. A common side effect of pain medications is constipation.

In the event that someone overdoses, the medication can be reversed with another medication called naloxone or Narcan. This will reverse the effects of fentanyl, but must be done cautiously. Withdrawal seizures can occur in patients who have been on the medicine for a long time.

WHAT ELSE SHOULD I DO? It is important to follow the instructions of your health care provider when taking this and similar medications. Over the years, clinicians have developed a great deal of experience in prescribing and monitoring the effects of medications such as fentanyl. Be sure to gain a clear understanding prior to using the product. As always, in the event that you have questions, seek appropriate medical advice.

fibromyalgia

I spoke at a local Senior Center on a variety of health care issues and an attendee asked me to write about Fibromyalgia, as a family member is afflicted with this medical condition. In the emergency department, a large percentage of our patients with acute and chronic pain that requires treatment. Many times, these patients suffer from Fibromyalgia and their pain needs to be addressed. .

WHAT IS FIBROMYALGIA? This is a chronic pain condition that involves the connective tissues including muscles, ligaments, and tendons. A patient may experience diffuse muscle type pain that is referred to as myalgia. There may be other associated problems such as generalized fatigue, headaches, sleep disturbances, depression, anxiety and mood swings.

This condition was first reported in France and England in the nineteenth century and was referred to as fibrositis, which means inflammation. Now, the term is better described with the suffix of "-algia" which means pain.

WHO IS AFFECTED? The medical literature has shown that women are more often afflicted with this disease (6:1), with a peak from ages 55 to 79. It is estimated that about 4 percent of American women suffer from some form of fibromyalgia. Yet, this can be seen in all age groups. One study has shown that 1 to 2 percent of young school age children hold the diagnosis.

WHAT ARE THE SYMPTOMS? The most common presentation is that of diffuse, generalized muscle-type pains. The pain may feel like a deep muscle pain that is consistent with aching, burning, stiffness or throbbing. Some patients may complain of a crawling sensation in the legs and arms.

The intensity of the pain may be varied and dependent on a variety of factors. Those factors may include stress, exposure to cold, insomnia, weather changes and exertion. Many feel worse in the morning with the condition improving as the day wears on.

The pain may be localized to a specific area which most often involves the upper body such as the neck and arms. But, this pain may involve other body parts. Some patients may report that the joints feel swollen, yet it is not obvious during the clinical examination.

PAIN

It is important to note that despite generalized symptoms being present, the diagnosis of fibromyalgia involves some very specific criterion set forth by the American College of Rheumatology (www.rheumatology.org).

WHAT ARE THE CAUSES? The exact cause of the disease is currently unknown. Research has shown that a variety of physical and emotional factors may trigger a flare. One study has looked at being infected with the Epstein-Barr virus as a causative factor.

There are other factors that may lead to generalized muscle pain. One of the most common seen is in patients who take the statin type cholesterol medications. Other medical conditions may include an inactive thyroid such as hypothyroidism and other forms of arthritis. It is important that your health provider assess all of these issues when working up the cause for muscle pain.

HOW IS THIS DIAGNOSED? Many patients suffer for several years prior to undergoing a workup. The health care provider will assess a patient's history and perform a variety of laboratory studies in order to rule out other medical problems. When this is done, the rheumatology "tender points" list will be assessed and if 11 of the 18 are met, the diagnosis is made.

WHAT IS THE TREATMENT? The treatment for this complicated medical problem will involve a variety of physician specialists, therapists and mental health care professionals. Some medications prescribed may include nonsteroidal anti-inflammatory drugs like ibuprofen, narcotics, antidepressants and antiseizure medications. All of these medications are used in chronic pain management and have been shown to be effective.

A variety of physical type modalities are used as well. This may include stress reduction, hypnotherapy, biofeedback and behavioral therapy. It has been shown that about half of all patients respond quite nicely to this conventional type of treatment.

This is a very complicated problem that requires significant medical investigation. Appropriate medical workup and treatment may improve the quality of life of the patient. In addition, your community may have local support groups that will assist the patient in living with the problem.

kidney stones

It seems that a day does not go by in the emergency department without some-one coming in with severe abdominal pain. The pain can be the worst ever ex-perienced in a person's life. It may be located in the back and in the abdominal area. This presentation is very common and the culprit may be a kidney stone.

WHAT IS A KIDNEY STONE? A kidney stone is a hard and firm mass that is very small and develops within the kidney. The kidney stone is about as big as the ball on a ballpoint pen and it may look like a sand burr when viewed under the microscope. To the patient, it feels like it is the size of a boulder!

The presence of kidney stones is referred to as nephrolithiasis in the kidney and urolithiasis when the stones are in the urinary tract. Usually, when the stones are in the ureter (the tube that brings urine down from the kidney to the bladder), the patient feels the most pain. The stone blocks the passage of urine, causing a backup and pressure.

WHAT CAUSES KIDNEY STONES? The exact cause for the formation of kidney stones is not completely known. It has been shown that crystals in the urine begin to stick together leading to the formation of the stone. This may be due to the lack of certain urine chemicals within the kidney.

It has been shown that a majority of kidney stones have calcium oxalate or cal-cium phosphate present in their composition. Some other types of stones may be secondary to infection in the urine or gout, which is an excess of uric acid in the body. No matter what type of stone, all are painful!

It has been thought that kidney stones may be caused by dehydration and many patients become symptomatic after the summer months. This is only a theory, but it is important to remain hydrated. In addition, it is known that patients tak-ing diuretics (water pills) are at risk for developing kidney stones.

WHO GETS KIDNEY STONES? There is a hereditary predisposition for the development of kidney stones. They are common in people ages 20 to 50. Men are more frequently affected– three times more than women. This is one of the most painful conditions a male will ever experience!

PAIN

WHAT ARE THE SYMPTOMS? Patients may experience some ongoing urinary symptoms prior to a full-blown attack by a kidney stone. They may complain of some urinary difficulty, pain or blood in the urine. Other people may just have a very sudden onset of back and abdominal pain that may radiate to the groin. The pain may be so severe, that the person may be nauseated and vomit. The pain may be rather sharp and stabbing. It may also come and go as well. It is unusual for a fever to be present, unless this is a chronic, untreated problem.

WHAT IS THE TREATMENT? In general, most initial presentations of a kidney stone are diagnosed and treated in the emergency department. The pain needs to be addressed with a shot of a narcotic and possibly a nonsteroidal anti-inflammatory drug like Toradol. Once the pain is under control, the patient needs to be examined and the urine must be analyzed for the presence of blood or infection. Usually an x-ray study will confirm the diagnosis. A high speed CT scan can be completed to show the location of the stone and the severity of the blockage.

In general, most patients are sent home with pain medication and told to strain their urine. When the stone passes in the urine and it is collected, the composition can be analyzed. A consultation with a urologist is usually in order as well. If the stone does not pass, it may need to be removed surgically.

Stones in the kidney may be broken up by lithrotripsy, which is a special ultrasound type of procedure. This usually makes the stones very small and they pass down the ureter without difficulty.

WHAT ELSE SHOULD BE DONE? If you have had a kidney stone in the past, you are at risk for another. You may need to alter your diet and medications. Most importantly, a consultation with a urologist will be able to help you make the necessary lifestyle changes.

sciatica

In our lifetime, we will all experience at least one episode of back pain. This is a very common condition that I see daily in the emergency department. A majority of the cases are quite straightforward and respond to a simple course of anti-inflammatory and pain relievers. These folks are sent home with some of these medications and in a week a two, they are back to baseline.

For others, the course may be much more complicated. The conservative treatment may fail and further intervention may be necessary. Recently, I experienced this first hand with my father, who is in his mid-seventies. He has been very active all his life and in retirement works at my hospital as a lab courier. My dad was getting out of a commercial airliner, when he had a sudden onset of some back pain with radiation down his leg. He was initially treated conservatively by his doctors for sciatica, but went on for surgical intervention.

WHAT IS SCIATICA? The sciatic nerve is a large nerve that runs down the middle of the leg. When the nerve becomes irritated or entrapped, pain will occur down the leg. The pain may be sharp or burning. It may run down the entirety of the leg, but it may be isolated to knee, ankle and foot pain.

The sciatic nerve comes out of the lower back, travels through the buttocks, down the thigh, calf and foot. Thus, a wide range of the leg can be affected. Usually, only one side may become irritated. The pain may come on rather suddenly. There may be some weakness in the leg that can be noticed while walking. The pain may become progressive throughout the day and worsened by standing.

With my dad, as his condition worsened, he had severe thigh pain. He went from walking several miles per day to being able to only walk from one chair to the next, and then having to sit down. This is very characteristic of sciatic nerve irritation.

WHAT CAUSES SCIATICA? There may be several conditions that lead to irritation of the nerve. In a majority of cases in younger individuals, about 85 percent of the time the cause is unknown. With older individuals, arthritis of the back is a leading cause. There may be spurs and narrowing of the joint space. A disc may be bulging or herniated. This is what is classically referred to as a "slipped disc."

PAIN

The other causes include muscle/ligament injuries and spinal stenosis. Spinal stenosis is a narrowed canal that carries the spinal cord. All of these conditions may irritate the nerve and lead to debilitating leg pain.

HOW IS SCIATICA DIAGNOSED? As with most medical conditions, an evaluation by a health care professional is in order. The history of the disease process and physical examination will lead to the diagnosis. Usually, in fairly straightforward cases, no blood work will be necessary. Plain x-rays may show some arthritic changes. A CT scan will be of little value. The test yielding the most information is the MRI. This x-ray will look internally at the boney and soft tissue structures. Arthritis and disc herniations will be quite obvious.

WHAT IS THE TREATMENT? Once the diagnosis is made, conservative management will be ordered. This may include the use of anti-inflammatory medications and narcotics. Physical therapy may be ordered. If that does not help, an epidural steroid injection may be given. This is a specialized shot in the back with a steroid.

With my dad, all of the conservative treatments failed. He was evaluated for an open surgical procedure, as well as an endoscopic surgery. Both procedures were to remove part of the disc that was pinching the nerve in the spinal canal. He opted for the endoscopic procedure by a very qualified spine surgeon. The surgery was completed through a very small incision in the back that did not even require stitches!

The most amazing part of the process was to see him hobble into the hospital on the morning of the surgery and literally walk out of the hospital a few hours later. Surgical intervention is not for everyone, and your doctor must carefully determine whether you will benefit the most from the procedure.

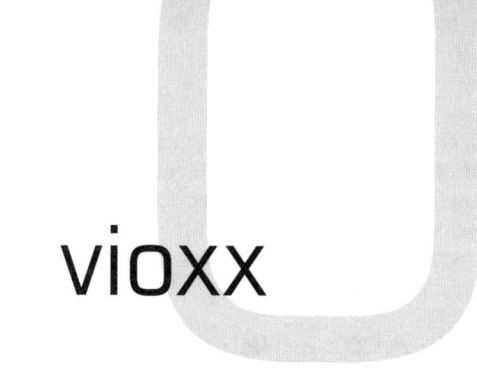

VIOXX

Vioxx, a very common pain reliever and anti-inflammatory drug, was voluntarily pulled from the market. This move was generated by the manufacturer, Merck Pharmaceuticals, despite the fact that over 2 million patients are taking this medication worldwide and that Merck had enjoyed over $2.5 billion in sales annually. Vioxx is a drug within the class of COX-2 inhibitors that are used for the treatment of osteoarthritis, rheumatoid arthritis and certain pain conditions.

WHY WAS THIS DRUG REMOVED? A study looked at the effects of Vioxx versus a placebo (sugar pill) on the development of recurrent colon polyps. Colon polyps are small growths of tissue within the colon that can be cancerous. Over the years, it has been shown that aspirin has decreased the incidence of colon cancer and polyps. Since aspirin and Vioxx are very similar, it was thought that Vioxx might decrease the incidence of re-developing colon polyps.

The study looked at a couple of questions– whether the Vioxx affected the rates of colon cancer and the long-term safety of using Vioxx. For the first 18 months of the study, there were no concerns about long-term usage. But it was noted that after 18 months, the risk of heart attack and stroke nearly doubled in those taking Vioxx.

According to the study, the chance of a heart attack or stroke in these patients not using Vioxx was about 75 percent. In the Vioxx group, the risk of heart attack or stroke was about 1.5 percent over that same time period.

Overall, Merck is being very cautious dealing with this information and safety concerns. Many physicians have felt that this recall was somewhat of an over-reaction. Of interest, numerous law firms have set up websites seeking patients who feel that they have been injured from the use of this drug.

WHAT IS A COX-2 INHIBITOR? The process of pain and inflammation is directed by a body chemical called cyclooxygenase, which occurs in two forms, 1 and 2. Over the years, health care providers have prescribed non-steroidal anti-inflammatory drugs (NSAIDS) like ibuprofen and naprosyn to treat pain and inflammation. The problem with these drugs is the possibility of developing stomach ulcers leading to bleeding. They also can contribute to changes in the blood and cause kidney failure. Even though they can be purchased over the counter, they must be used with caution.

PAIN

The COX-2 inhibitors were developed as more specific drugs that had less chance of developing bleeding in the gastrointestinal system. There have been three on the market known as Vioxx, Celebrex and Bextra. All three medications have been successful in treating pain from arthritis. The benefit has been a decreased chance of developing a stomach ulcer. Several medical studies have supported this claim.

WHY TAKE A COX-2 INHIBITOR? For patients affected with various types of arthritis and pain conditions, it is essential that their pain be managed daily with minimal side effects. It has been shown that these drugs have provided good pain control, less effects on the blood compatibility with Coumadin, and less chance of worsening asthma conditions. It is well known that aspirin-like drugs can worsen asthma.

WHAT SHOULD I DO? If you are taking Vioxx, you must contact your health care provider to discuss your options. The chance of side effects noted in the study with Vioxx were small, so do not panic! Your clinician will determine if you need a switch to Celebrex, Bextra or another medication. You will not be able to refill your Vioxx, so you must seek medical advice. There is no risk to suddenly discontinuing Vioxx.

As you wait to see your provider, you can access additional information at www.merck.com, www.vioxx.com. or by calling 888.36VIOXX.

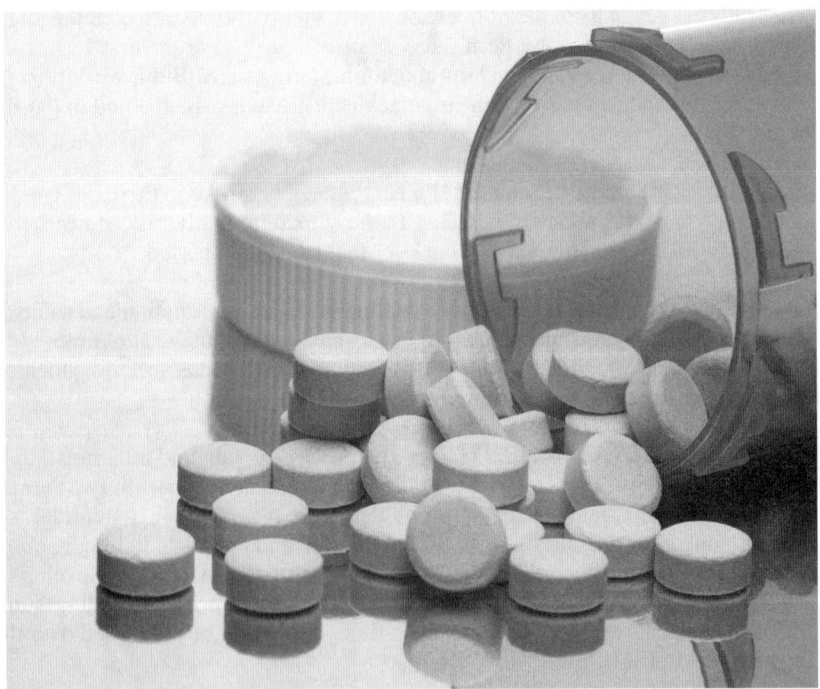

child
obesity

As the fast food industry has successfully "Supersized" their meals and bank-rolls, they have done the same for the American body, both young and old. Our nation has become 20 percent heavier in the past decade and some health experts have deemed this a pandemic—a widespread epidemic of illness. It not only affects our health, but the airline industry has had to recently recalculate weight loads that an airplane can handle! Our nation is headed for a health care crisis, with obesity being a major cause of several debilitating and life-threatening ill-nesses.

HOW IS OBESITY DEFINED? Obesity is defined as an excess of body fat mass. There are numerous ways that this can be determined, but a simple way is to calculate Body Mass Index (BMI). This can be determined by using a chart or done on your own using a proven formula. If you wish to calculate this on your own, multiply your weight in pounds by 703. This number should then be divided by your height in inches, two times.

A BMI of less than 25 is normal, 25-30 indicates that one is overweight, and greater than 30 indicates obesity. Medical studies have shown that patients with a BMI greater than 30 have an increased risk for several health problems.

IS THERE AN OBESITY PANDEMIC IN AMERICA? Yes! Overall, Americans are at least 20 percent heavier than they were in the 1980s. A major health care issue is the increase in obesity in our youth. American youth's rate of obesity has increased 25 percent in the past 10 years. Pediatricians have be-gun to focus on this health maintenance issue because unfortunately, this weight gain in children and adolescents has translated into a weight gain as adults.

Recent studies have shown that obese 10 to 13 year olds have an 80 percent chance of becoming obese adults. This has tremendous health implications for our adult population.

WHAT ARE THE RISKS OF OBESITY? It has been clearly defined in medical literature that obese individuals are at risk for other health problems. This includes diabetes, high cholesterol, high blood pressure, heart disease, sleep disturbances, arthritis and poor quality of life. Many of these diseases are major risk factors for the development of heart disease.

PEDIATRICS

WHAT CAN I DO? It is important to realize that overweight children may turn into overweight adults. We need to develop healthy eating habits in our children and youth and show them the importance of a healthy diet.

A well-balanced diet includes balanced portions of protein, carbohydrates and fats. Food high in sugar content, such as sodas and fruit drinks, should be discouraged. Eating habits should be monitored and frequent snacking avoided.

In addition, exercise is essential in the prevention of obesity. Studies have shown that children of parents that exercise also develop those healthy exercise habits. Parents need to set good examples for their children by maintaining an active lifestyle. Encourage children to participate in physical activities and athletics, and limit the time they spend in front of the television, video games and computer.

HOW CAN WE HELP OUR YOUTH? As adults, we need to create a healthy home food-environment. Reduce the consumption of fast foods by limiting this to a maximum of one time per week. Encourage the consumption of water over soft drinks. Provide appropriate food portions so that "cleaning one's plate" is a viable goal. It is also important to educate children on healthy foods and alternatives to candies and sweets.

In addition to good eating, encourage children to be physically active. Create an environment for active play inside and outside the home. Limit television and computer time to a couple hours per week. Provide physical activity alternatives on a daily basis and reserve a weekend day for some physical activity.

Overall, providing a safe and healthy environment for children will help them develop good habits for a lifetime. These simple steps may help us reverse the unfortunate trend of increasing weight, obesity and chronic preventable diseases.

conjoined twins

When a couple first finds out that they are expecting a child, many things go through their minds. Will it be a boy or girl? Will the pregnancy go all right? How big will the baby be? And, most importantly, parents focus on the health of their child. Imagine then, when you are at your doctor's office and you are told that you are carrying twins, but there is a complication. They are conjoined. Your immediate thoughts turn to where they are conjoined, if this can be fixed and how people will accept them.

WHAT ARE CONJOINED TWINS? Conjoined twins, previously referred to as Siamese twins, are individuals that are born attached to each other. These twins are identical twins that develop from a single fertilized ovum and develop in a single placenta. They are always the same sex and the same race. In terms of gender, it is three times more common in females than males.

HOW COMMON IS THIS? This may occur once in every 40,000 births, but only once in every 200,000 live births. About 40 to 60 percent of these sets of twins are delivered stillborn, and only 35 percent survive for one day. The overall survival rate for conjoined twins is anywhere from 5 to 25 percent. In the United States, there are a few sets of surviving conjoined twins.

History has documented about 600 sets of conjoined twins in the past 500 years that have survived. The largest number of these twins are in India and Africa. There are no documented cases of conjoined triplets or quadruplets.

HOW DOES THIS OCCUR? As a developing embryo begins to split to form identical twins within the first two weeks after conception, the splitting process ceases. This leaves a partially separated egg that develops into a mature conjoined fetus. The process may be influenced by environmental and genetic factors. It is thought that the failure of the twins to split occurs on day 13 after fertilization.

WHAT ARE THE TYPES OF CONJOINED TWINS? The classification of the twins is based on the point of attachment. The Greek word, pagos "that which is fixed," is used to describe the twins. There are three-dozen types based on this classification scheme.

PEDIATRICS

Twins joined at the head are referred to as craniopagus. Only two percent of all cases are joined at the head. Pygopagus twins are joined at the rump and account for 19 percent of all cases. Both of these types do not share the heart or umbilicus (bellybutton).

There are several midline conjoined twin classifications that involve the umbilicus. This may include a variety of attachments of the trunk or lower half of the body. The most common conjoined twin is joined in the upper trunk and they usually share the same heart.

The most famous set of twins were Chang and Eng Bunker who were born in 1811 and died in 1874, at the age of 63. They were joined at the abdomen. They were born in Thailand, but lived in North Carolina. They married sisters and fathered 21 children. They were successful businessmen and ranchers. Their lives were quite private, but they did earn a great deal of money touring the world.

WHAT CAN BE DONE? Medical specialists have been confronted with these issues over the years. Successful surgical separations date back to the 1950s. It is necessary to assemble a multispecialty team in order to deal with the situation. The surgery is usually very complicated and requires a great deal of preparation. Throughout the years, several successful surgical separations have been accomplished on very young twins.

fructose intolerance

Over the years, we have become more and more aware of food intolerances and allergies. Airlines and schools have altered their menus. Restaurants disclose their ingredients. Lawsuits have ensued after serious reactions to various food groups.

A little known food problem is fructose intolerance. Fructose is a form of sugar found in a variety of fruits and other sweet foods. In the United States, about 1 person in 20,000 suffers from this disease formally known as Fructose Intolerance.

WHAT IS FRUCTOSE INTOLERANCE? This is a metabolic problem in which a person is unable to digest fructose, a sugar found in fruits, or sucrose—which is common table sugar. In 1956 it was found that these individuals lack an important enzyme called Aldolase B. An enzyme is a body chemical that helps break down foods or works as a helper in other chemical reactions.

When the body is unable to digest sugars, there is inadequate blood sugar available in the body and the patient experiences hypoglycemia, known as low blood sugar. This is a serious, life-threatening problem. In addition, when the fructose and sucrose are not broken down, they are deposited in the liver. This eventually leads to liver failure and eventual death if untreated.

WHAT ARE THE SYMPTOMS? Fructose Intolerance is a recessive hereditary disease. Thus, it may not always be obvious that this is the problem. Usually, an infant may experience symptoms after being fed fruits early in their diet or a child may experience symptoms after eating soy formula. The child may not eat very well and become irritable. They may be lethargic and sleep a lot. Parents may notice that there are no symptoms if fruits are removed from the diet. Severe cases may include nausea and vomiting.

If left untreated, liver problems may become present. The child may be jaundiced, which is a yellow color noted on skin and the whites of the eyes. Jaundice comes from bilirubin, a breakdown product in the liver. The liver may also be enlarged and can be felt on physical exam.

PEDIATRICS

HOW IS THIS DIAGNOSED? If there is a family history of this problem, the health care provider must be suspicious of this disease. Next, a dietary history is essential and symptoms should be noted when exposed to fructose and sucrose. Elimination of the sugars from the diet and a resultant absence of symptoms helps in the diagnostic process.

The physical examination may lend clues to the diagnosis with the findings noted above. A variety of laboratory tests will confirm the diagnosis, which include chemical abnormalities in the urine. In addition, a controlled test may include monitoring blood sugar level after fructose or sucrose is ingested. If positive, a patient will become hypoglycemic after eating sugars, which is the opposite of what is normally expected.

Additional testing will include assessment of the liver through blood tests. In severe and late stage disease, a liver biopsy may be necessary. Finally, enzyme studies on the blood and genetic studies can be completed to confirm the disease. It should be noted that these patients are also at risk for gout, which is a problem with uric acid. Thus, this must be assessed as well.

WHAT IS THE TREATMENT? Once the diagnosis is made, fructose and sucrose must be avoided. This is the mainstay of treatment and the patient can lead a fairly normal life. In addition, other medical conditions such as gout should be addressed to prevent other medical complications.

The prognosis for this disease is excellent, once diagnosis is made. Appropriate dietary modifications are essential. If there is evidence of liver disease, this will slowly improve and resolve with appropriate avoidance of sugars. Most common complications are low blood sugar, liver failure and other organ damage. But, when treated, life expectancy is normal.

If there is a family history of this problem, children should be screened by a genetic specialist. A team approach to care with a child should involve the pediatrician and a dietician. This will lead to a full and healthy life. Most importantly, if there is concern about this disease, prompt medical attention is essential.

pediatric poisoning

In 2003, the American Academy of Pediatrics issued a new policy statement on the home treatment of poisoning in children. The recommendations that have been in place for over 30 years have changed. Prevention of accidental poisonings and the initial home treatment recommendations have been significantly altered.

In the United States, there are over one million cases of accidental pediatric poisonings. Fortunately, the consequences of these incidents have not been as severe as in recent years. In the 1940s, over 500 children died annually after a poisoning event. At present, less than 25 childhood deaths occur each year after accidental ingestion.

Over the years, there has been increased attention addressed at the prevention of childhood poisonings. In addition, many of the toxic household drugs have been replaced with safer drugs and there has been a greater focus on the development of poison control centers.

WHAT SHOULD BE DONE IF MY CHILD IS POISONED? The initial first aid measures for poisoning involve initially protecting your child from further injury. In the event that the exposure is serious, call 911 and seek immediate medical attention. Be sure to have as much information available for the emergency medical providers as possible– including containers and bottles of the offending substance.

In the event that the ingestion can be treated at home, it is important to contact the **Poison Control Center at (800) 222-1222**. This is a national number that will route your call to a local state agency. Poison Control Centers are staffed 24 hours daily by toxicology technicians and toxicologists.

You will be given appropriate instructions on how to deal with the home emergency. You will also be told if it is necessary to seek immediate medical attention. If you need to visit your emergency department, the Poison Control Center usually notifies the emergency department staff of the impending visit and treatment recommendations.

PEDIATRICS

WHAT ARE THE NEW RECOMMENDATIONS FOR
TREATMENT? Since the 1960s, Ipecac has been available as an over-the-counter medication that induces vomiting. It has been shown over the years that it was important to remove the poison from a child's stomach by using this medicine. Once given, a child will start vomiting within about 20 minutes. This has been thought to clear the stomach of the offending poison. Recent research has not supported the home use of Ipecac or Activated Charcoal. Activated Charcoal is given in the emergency department in order to absorb poisons in the child's stomach.

Recent research has questioned the safety and effectiveness of Ipecac. It has now been shown that Ipecac can be dangerous and the risks outweigh the benefits. Some problems with Ipecac have included the possibility of aspirating the vomitus into the lungs, sleepiness and the inability for the child to tolerate oral antidotes or absorptive medicines. With corrosive substances, making a child vomit these back up will cause additional damage to the body.

WHAT ELSE CAN I DO? First, remain calm and call Poison Control. Gather as much information as possible to help your health care providers and then seek medical attention. Basic first aid measures should be implemented such as maintaining an open airway, checking breathing, and monitoring circulation. Be sure to utilize your pre-hospital emergency care providers if needed.

Prevention is the most important step. Keep poisons and medicines out of the reach of children. Be sure to engage childproof safety caps on containers. Never transfer poisonous substances or medications from their original containers. Be sure to properly dispose of old chemicals and medicines. Never refer to medicines as "candy" to children, because this is the setting for disaster!

It is now recommended that you properly dispose of Ipecac that you may have in your medicine cabinet. You should no longer give this medicine under any circumstances, unless directed by you doctor. If stomach decontamination is necessary, it must be done under the supervision of medical professionals in the hospital.

To Your Health with Dr. Wojo

scoliosis

Scoliosis is often discovered during a child's annual or biannual examination. This is a fairly common problem that needs to be addressed, so let's look a little more closely at scoliosis.

WHAT IS SCOLIOSIS? Scoliosis is a curvature of the spine. Instead of the spine being in a straight line, it is bent from side to side. The bones of the back are called the vertebrae. The neck bones are called cervical vertebrae and the midback bones are the thoracic vertebrae. The "small of the back" vertebrae compose the lumbar spine. All of these bones should stack upon each other in a straight line. Normal curves of the spine will be forward and back.

With scoliosis, the most commonly involved area is the thoracic spine. There are 12 thoracic vertebrae, so this involves a fairly large area. The bones of the "small of the back" are rarely involved, as are the neck bones.

WHAT CAUSES SCOLIOSIS? There are many causes for scoliosis, but 80 to 85 percent of the cases are called idiopathic. This means that there is no known cause and it just happens. Usually, scoliosis will develop gradually over time and is more pronounced as a child develops. That is why the sports physical may be the first time that this condition is detected. Sometimes, parents may notice a change in their child's posture and alert their health care provider to the condition.

Nonstructural or functional scoliosis is seen when the normal spine appears curved and the condition may be temporary. The temporary causes may be due to a muscle spasm or a shortened leg. Once the temporary cause is corrected, the spine returns to its normal configuration.

Structural scoliosis is when the spine is fixed in an abnormal curve. There is usually an underlying medical problem that may be caused by a tissue disorder, arthritis, cerebral palsy, polio, birth defect or tumor. But it is important to remember that a majority of these cases have no known cause.

PEDIATRICS

WHAT ARE THE SYMPTOMS? Usually, a child or teenager may have no complaints of pain, but just a noticeable deformity. The shoulders may seem uneven or a shoulder blade may be sticking out. There may be an obvious curve in the back or a hump. Eventually, it may be noticeable that the person is leaning to one side and this may lead to back pain.

HOW IS IT DIAGNOSED? Diagnosis is made on the basis of the history of the patient and physical examination by a health care provider. The spine may be x-rayed to evaluate the spine in a more precise manner. Usually, the sports physical is a time when this screening may occur.

WHO IS AT RISK? Usually girls are affected more often than boys. Young children with scoliosis will magnify the curve as they grow. Lastly, children that are born with a spinal abnormality are at increased risk for problems as they grow.

WHAT IS THE TREATMENT? Initially, the diagnosis must be made and then the progression must be watched. Many children will outgrow this, but it must be closely observed. Early diagnosis leads to a better outcome if more aggressive therapy is necessary. Checkups are usually recommended every 3 to 6 months.

Initial medical treatment may involve wearing a brace. One of the most common braces is called the Milwaukee brace, which helps stop the progression of the curve. This is the only option during the growing years and it essential that it is worn prior to the cessation of the growth spurt. This is a fairly successful method of treatment.

If bracing does not stop the development of the curve or the scoliosis is caught too late, surgery may be necessary. The surgical procedure may involve the placement of a rod in the spine to stop the curve from worsening. Sometimes, the vertebrae are fused together as well. Some nonconventional treatment methods have no proven success in the medical literature. Be careful to stick with proven medical and surgical methods.

spina bifida

It seems that the news from the Iraq War is not always positive, but a humanitarian act by the military drew our attention. While on patrol, army forces discovered a four-month-old baby that had a birth defect and had received inadequate medical care. The defect was spina bifida—a condition where the child's spinal column had not properly fused, thus exposing the spinal cord.

The military made a plea to the United States government to bring the child to America for treatment. Doctors at Children's Healthcare of Atlanta volunteered their services and Baby Noor underwent successful surgery to close the defect in her back. She will never be able to walk, but she can have a fruitful life.

Spina Bifida is fairly rare, but not unheard of in the United States. Let's take a closer look at the issues surrounding this birth defect and current treatment options.

WHAT IS SPINA BIFIDA? This birth defect occurs during the first month of pregnancy when the spinal column does not close in the small of the back, leaving the baby with an exposed spinal column. In the United States there are about 70,000 people living with spinda bifida and about 3,000 babies are born each year with this spinal column defect.

There are varying cases of severity of spina bifida. Brain damage may be present, as well as damage to the outer covering of the spinal cord. Exposed nerves in the lower back will be damaged and the affected person will not be able to walk. In addition, some patients may have brain damage including hydrocephalus—increased fluid on the brain. Other complications may include bowel and bladder trouble.

WHO IS AT RISK? Research has shown that children of mothers of low socioeconomic status are at risk. Caucasians are at greater risk. Mothers with a seizure disorder taking antiseizure medications present a greater risk. Insulin dependent diabetes in the mother also increases the risk. A previous pregnancy with a neural tube defect increases the risk, by 20 times, that a subsequent pregnancy will be affected. Exposure to a high fever during pregnancy has also been shown to increase the chances of a fetus being affected. Most of these factors cannot be controlled.

PEDIATRICS

WHAT IS THE TREATMENT? There is no cure for spina bifida because skin, nerve, and bone cannot be replaced. But, as with Baby Noor, surgical intervention is used to close the defect in the back and protect the spinal column. Other medical problems associated with spina bifida can be corrected, such as structural abnormalities in the bladder and the bowel. The sooner the surgical intervention, the better, as the risk of infection is markedly decreased if correction occurs within the first 24 hours of life.

Other issues, including brain damage from hydrocephalus, must be addressed if present. A shunt may be surgically placed to relieve pressure in the brain. This occurs in the most severe cases, but not with Baby Noor.

Most children that are appropriately treated will lead a productive life into adulthood. Medication may be necessary to address some problems. Most importantly, aggressive physical and occupational therapy needs to be provided. Lastly, a combination of wheelchairs and bracing will lead to good mobility.

WHAT IS THE PROGNOSIS? With early intervention, the prognosis is good. A patient will be able to live into adulthood with minimal difficulty. Granted, if there are numerous physical abnormalities, the chances of survival are not as great.

WHAT IS THE CURRENT RESEARCH? The National Institutes of Neurological Disorders and Stroke (NINDS) continue to conduct studies into the causes of spina bifida. Research is aimed at preventing, treating and curing the disorder. Recent studies have shown that the addition of .40 mg folic acid to a pregnant woman's dietary regimen, can reduce the occurrence and incidence of neural tube defects that lead to the development of spina bifida. This is essential and a very simple task to complete on a daily basis.

If you wish to learn more about the disease and associated support groups, go to http://www.ninds.nih.gov/ for further information.

sudden infant death syndrome
(SIDS)

For years, medical professionals have been perplexed by cases of apparently healthy infants dying in their sleep—known as Sudden Infant Death Syndrome (SIDS). Even though researchers are not close to solving the problem, they have gleaned more information about this complex situation and some of the risk factors. It is important to be aware of these risk factors in order to decrease the incidence of SIDS.

WHAT IS SIDS? SIDS is defined as the sudden and unexpected death of an infant that is usually under the age of one. The average age of a SIDS victim is six months. Death is attributed to SIDS after a thorough investigation reveals no underlying medical pathology and an examination of the scene and the family history are completed.

A similar problem is referred to as sudden unexpected death in infancy, which is referred to as SUDI. SUDI has a defined cause of death such as suffocation, accidental poisoning, falls, respiratory illness, child abuse or homicide. These deaths may be identified during a SIDS investigation.

IS THIS A COMMON PROBLEM? In the United States, there are about 3,000 SIDS deaths each year. Fortunately since 1990, the death rate in the United States has declined by nearly 50 percent. SIDS is the third leading cause of infant mortality overall, but it is the leading cause of death in infants in their first year of life.

WHAT ARE THE CAUSES? A single cause for SIDS is unknown. A study at the University of Washington identified a higher level of the male hormone known as testosterone in infants that had died. It is known that higher levels of testosterone will suppress a respiratory drive in adults. Researchers investigating this hypothesis found that SIDS victims, both male and female, had higher than normal testosterone levels upon autopsy evaluation. The clinical utility of this information needs to be further determined.

It is known that infants are at risk during a certain developmental window. Postmortem evaluation of SIDS victims has noted some changes in the infant's brain. The areas of the brain involved may help stimulate the breathing process. Once again, continued investigation into this information is warranted.

PEDIATRICS

WHAT ARE THE RISK FACTORS? Identifying risk factors and making the public aware of them is of the utmost importance. It is known that babies born to mothers under the age of 20 are at risk—especially so if the mother did not receive pre-natal care. Drug abuse and smoking during pregnancy have been shown to increase the chance for SIDS. An infant that is exposed to smoking while in-utero and after birth is a significant risk for SIDS. These are definitely controllable factors.

Research has shown that infant risk factors include prone or side sleeping, especially on soft surfaces with loose bedding. For years, it was thought that a child must sleep on their belly, as there was concern about spitting up and choking. This is not the case. Also, infants should not sleep in waterbeds, on a sofa, or with stuffed toys.

WHAT ARE THE RECOMMENDATIONS TO PREVENT SIDS?
Mothers must not smoke during pregnancy and the child must not be exposed to smoke after birth. Exposure to smoking after birth has been shown to increase the incidence of respiratory illnesses. Infants must sleep on their backs and loose bedding must be removed. The infant must not become overheated and should not share a bed. Pacifiers may help a child fall to sleep and do not increase the risk for SIDS.

In the past 15 years, great strides have been made to reduce the incidence of SIDS. We still do not know the specific causes for the development of the problem, but we are aware of the controllable risk factors. More information may be obtained through the American Sudden Infant Death Institute at www.sids.org.

bees

As summer comes to an end, wasps work overtime and that means more individuals visit the emergency department because of stings. There have been single stings and multiple stings with a variety of presentations that have required basic and aggressive treatment.

Each year, bees sting about one to two million Americans. This results in about one hundred deaths annually, but this may be under reported. Some of these individuals that die may have their cause of death ruled as a heart condition or an asthma attack. But, the inciting factor was a pesky bee.

PREVENTION IS BEST! It is best to avoid bees at all cost. Avoid bright colored clothing and perfumes because bees are attracted to this and they land to check it out. They are also attracted to sweat, so this places you at risk for a sting. When drinking a canned beverage outside, be careful as bees like to sneak inside!

Common sense is important. Wear shoes when walking through vegetation and working around the yard. Protective clothing will diminish your chance of being stung. Be aware where there are ground nests and avoid them. If you are attacked, you need to flee the scene. Bees emit a scent that attracts other bees to attack. If you are near water and it is safe, jump in. Otherwise, get into a building for protection.

WHAT SHOULD I DO IF STUNG? Do not panic! About one percent of all people stung by bees have experienced a true anaphylactic (severe allergic) reaction that requires immediate emergency attention. The rest of those affected require some first aid and medical treatment.

If an acute anaphylactic reaction occurs, call 911 and seek emergency treatment. These symptoms would include severe respiratory distress, throat swelling, facial swelling, low blood pressure, passing out and a severe rash. Emergency treatment will include protecting the airway, administration of epinephrine from an Epi-Pen, administration of antihistamines and steroids. Some patients may need to be admitted to the hospital for observation of severe symptoms.

A majority of cases do not require such aggressive treatment. Once the patient is in a safe environment, several things can be done. Removal of a remaining stinger is important, as bee venom may still be present in the stinger. It has always been recommended that the stinger be scraped off the skin and not removed with tweezers. Recent literature has shown that removal technique may not matter.

Next, apply ice to the swollen area to prevent progression of swelling in the involved area. It may be wise to take an antihistamine like diphenhydramine (Benadryl). This may slow down an allergic response.

Sometimes, an area may become infected and treatment with antibiotics may be necessary. This is usually not the case, but if concerned, have a health care provider assess the situation.

Some other home remedies have been listed on the Internet. This may include the use of meat tenderizer or ammonia applied directly to the wound. I have little experience with these home remedies and there is not a lot of medical literature available on the safety and success of these treatments. Thus, I do not recommend these modalities.

Usually, redness and swelling will go away in a few days when utilizing ice and antihistamines. If concerned, seek medical attention.

Most importantly, if you are allergic to bees, there is hope. Seek treatment from an allergist. Desensitization treatments are highly effective and successful. This involves a series of shots. This treatment will protect you from severe anaphylactic reactions and even death.

While you are in the process of seeking allergy treatment, you must carry an epi-pen with you at all times. This auto-injector has a dose of epinephrine or adrenaline that will stop a severe life-threatening allergic reaction. Be sure to always keep it with you during these high-risk times, as it may save your life.

boating safety

There are several simple things we can do to maintain safety while boating or participating in water sports. So, let's take a look at a few things that you can do to make the summer safer when you fire up the old boat motor and head out for some fun.

KNOW THE RULES. You must understand your local and state boating rules. In Wisconsin, your motorboat must be registered with the Department of Natural Resources and the registration must be renewed every couple of years. Be sure to have the registration handy and the registration numbers displayed properly with the renewal sticker.

My son completed the DNR boater's safety course. He was issued a certificate to operate a boat alone. This course must be completed so that children ages 12 to 15 may operate a boat by themselves. The course is excellent and provides a great deal of maritime information and general safety information.

Remember to have enough life vests on board. The law requires one per person and children ages 12 and under must wear a life jacket at all times while on the boat. This is good common sense and should apply to adults as well. A majority of the fatalities that are associated with boating are secondary to drowning. Be sure that the life vests are properly sized. For boats over 16 feet, there must be a throwable device on board.

KNOW YOUR BOAT. Studies have shown that a majority of boating accidents involve individuals who are unfamiliar with their craft and have not taken a boating safety course. A variety of things can go wrong with the boat, so be sure that it is adequately maintained. Passengers can be overcome by carbon monoxide poisoning, when sitting too close to the motor. If you develop a headache, nausea and fatigue, you may be a victim of this deadly gas. You will then need to be exposed to fresh air or even oxygen.

Be sure that all parts of the boat are functioning properly and stay away from the prop. I have seen some terrible injuries because people have gotten too close to the spinning prop. Permanent loss of a limb and even death can occur when one gets too close.

SEASONAL

It is important to operate the craft at prudent speeds, especially in unfamiliar waterways. The Wisconsin River can be a difficult place to navigate with many hidden dangers that can destroy your boat and your confidence and cause significant personal injury.

Since boats are powered by fuel, there is always a risk for fire. Motorboats must have a fire extinguisher on board. Take time to assess that it is properly charged and functioning. It is also important to know how to use the extinguisher, as there is no time to learn during a fire.

In the event of a fire, make sure everyone dons life vests and position the boat so that the fire is downwind. This will prevent further injury and smoke inhalation. Access the fire extinguisher and use it. There is a very simple principle referred to as PASS. Pull the pin. Aim at the fire. Squeeze the handle. Sweep from side to side. Burned passengers must seek immediate medical attention.

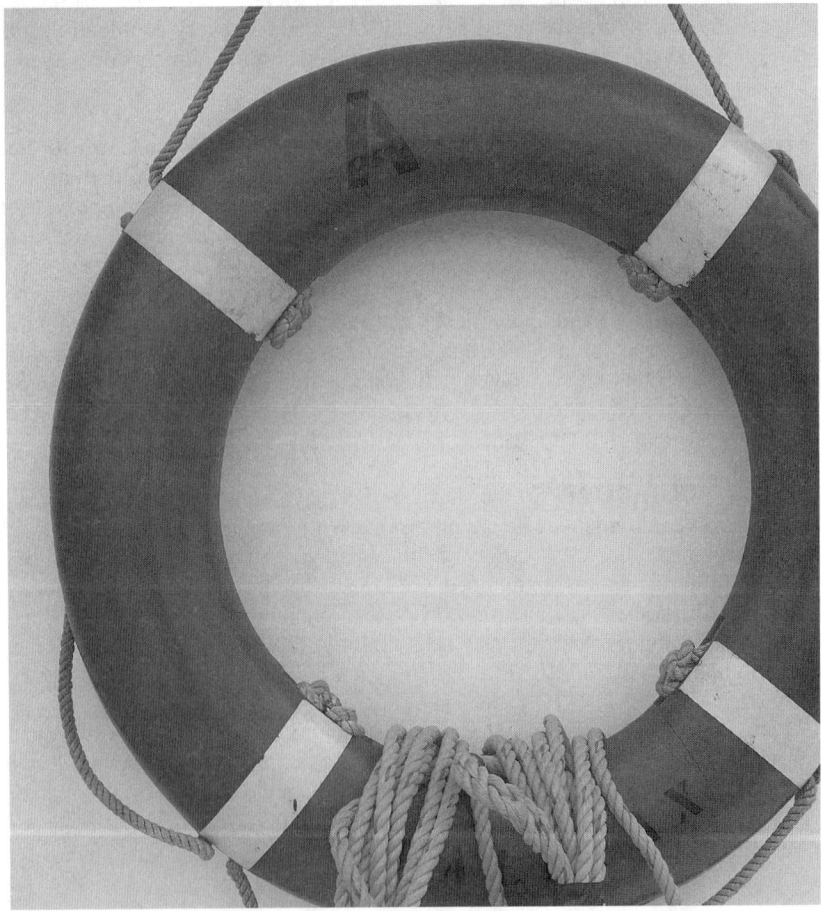

To Your Health with Dr. Wojo

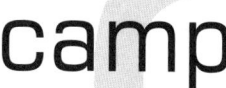

camp

In the United States, over 10 million children attend summer camp, and most camps have comprehensive medical and emergency plans in place. There are no federal requirements or guidelines mandated, but most camps must address these needs.

In addition to over 10 million campers, there are over one million camp counselors and administrators. The training can be varied, as the staff must attend to cuts, scrapes, vomiting, homesickness and more complicated problems such as diabetes or seizures.

In 2005, the American Academy of Pediatrics issued a very detailed set of guidelines that parents should evaluate when sending their son or daughter off to camp.

WHAT QUESTIONS DO I NEED TO ASK OF A CAMP? When first evaluating a camp, your choices may be directed by previous experience with a camp or based upon the recommendation of a family member or friend. Prior experience with a camp is very helpful, but a parent should still evaluate the camp thoroughly before making a decision.

When evaluating the medical and emergency procedures, ask to see the camp's written policies for dealing with medical emergencies and health issues. Written policies and protocols are essential, as this gives the counselors and staff members a consistent method for dealing with a crisis. You may wish to have a medical professional review the policies if you are concerned.

It is important to assess if the staff members are appropriately trained in emergency medical care such as first aid. Many large camps have nurses and physicians on staff. These medical professionals usually help in developing protocols and implementing them as well. They will usually help in training the staff prior to the arrival of campers.

You may wish to investigate/research the Emergency Medical Services System that is available to the camp. You need to know how quickly an ambulance can be dispatched and how long the transport time to the local medical facility will be. You may also want to assess the level of training of the emergency personnel as well. Feel free to visit the local ambulance provider, as they would be happy to show off their equipment.

HOW DO I PREPARE MY CHILD FOR CAMP? Most camps require a physical examination of the camper prior to admission to the camp. This is an excellent requirement, as children are screened for a variety of health care issues. Healthy children may have this examination within six months of arriving at camp, but camps may have their own requirements. Be sure to check on specific requirements.

It is essential that parents inform the camp of their child's medical problems, illnesses, injuries, surgeries and immunizations. Also, it is important to detail any mental health issues that have been treated prior to arrival at camp. Be sure that your child's immunizations are up-to-date and appropriately documented.

Most camps require extensive medical paperwork. Be sure to fill it out completely and accurately. Make sure that the consent for emergency treatment form is signed. Also, be sure to include all emergency contact phone numbers of several family members. It is frustrating for emergency medical professionals when family members cannot be reached in a time of crisis. Lastly, do not forget to include your health insurance information, as this will expedite the admission process at the hospital or clinic, if a visit is warranted.

When bringing medications to camp that need to be administered by the camp staff, be sure to bring those medications in their original containers with clearcut instructions. Most camps will not administer medications that have been removed from their original packaging, as this is an unsafe practice.

WHAT ELSE SHOULD I DO? A child's visit to summer camp is an invaluable adventure. Be sure that you assess the camp prior to arrival. Also, be sure that all of your child's medical information and medical needs are addressed prior to arrival. By following the above simple steps, both you and your child will have a great summer experience!

carbon monoxide

A SILENT KILLER IN YOUR HOME.

DR. WOJO'S PRESCRIPTION INSCRIPTION:
When your gas furnace goes on, your house will be warmed from the chill – but, be aware that carbon monoxide may be in the air, and your family it could kill!

Each year, as gas furnaces light up across the colder climates of the United States and warm our homes, our families are protected from the elements.

But unfortunately and tragically, this isn't always the case. In fact, some families are put at serious – even fatal – risk each cold weather season due to problems with their gas furnaces.

The cause is carbon monoxide, a silent killer in your home.

WHAT DO I NEED TO KNOW? Carbon monoxide is a colorless, odorless gas that is a by-product of combustion, the reaction that takes place within a motor. The most frequent source of carbon monoxide (CO) is a faulty furnace. The second most common source is an automobile. CO is also produced by a variety of other fuel-powered devices and heating sources that are extremely dangerous when used in poorly-ventilated areas.

During times of cooler weather, the risk of CO poisoning grows because furnaces are being switched on after sitting idle during warmer months. This is when furnaces are most likely to malfunction, which can result in CO poisoning.

HOW BAD IS IT? There are more than 40,000 visits each year to hospital emergency rooms because of CO poisonings, making it one of the most common forms of poisoning in America! Between 1,000 and 5,000 patients die, and countless others suffer from long-term disabilities as a result of CO exposure.

Tissue and organ damage can occur from oxygen starvation, and the chemical breakdown of CO in the body can cause brain damage. Of course, the worst-case scenario is, as happens far too often and needlessly, families go to sleep and never wake up!

SEASONAL

But CO poisoning isn't only a cold weather danger. Even during the warmer months, a person can be at risk for CO exposure from a faulty exhaust system on the car, or by working with gas-powered engines in poorly ventilated spaces.

WHAT ARE THE SYMPTOMS? There are no classic symptoms of CO poisoning. Recent studies have shown that nearly 25 percent of all patients may have a headache. Other symptoms may simply involve flu-like symptoms such as nausea, vomiting and "just not feeling well". More extreme symptoms can include severe nausea and vomiting, changes in mental status, seizures and even coma. The classic description of "cherry red" skin and mucous membranes is more unusual.

Helpful information to tell the doctor includes when the symptoms started; if any other family members have the same symptoms; and noticing if health improved when outside of the home or workplace.

Getting a proper diagnosis and the right care – as well as getting the CO problem fixed – is critical to your family's health. Tissue and organ damage can occur from oxygen starvation, and the chemical breakdown of CO in the body can cause brain damage. Of course, the worst-case scenario is, as happens far too often and needlessly, families go to sleep and never wake up!

WHAT IS THE TREATMENT? Emergency treatment for CO poisoning begins by moving the patient to a safe, well-ventilated area. Oxygen therapy is provided by the paramedics and continues in the hospital. The length of therapy depends on the levels of CO present in the blood and how quickly it is removed.

Over the years, treating CO poisoned patients in a hyperbaric oxygen chamber (which provides oxygen to the body under high pressure) has become more common. Medical studies have shown that patients suffering from severe CO poisoning benefit most from hyperbaric therapy. Long-term effects from CO poisoning — including problems with memory, concentration, depression and anxiety — have been notably reduced following this treatment.

WHAT CAN I DO? Have your furnace checked annually by a heating professional, and by all means, purchase CO detectors. Today, many smoke detectors also feature CO detectors, making them a great investment not only in dollars…but in sense! And remember, cut and save Dr. Wojo's Prescription Inscription.

cold & hypothermia

Cold hands and feet giving you the chills,
Hypothermia cannot be treated with pills.
Warm blankets and hats may be the key,
But sometimes you will leave with a hospital fee.

Each year, as the cooler winter months arrive, risk for cold-related injuries such as hypothermia increases. It does not always have to be very cold outside. Prolonged exposure may contribute to this significant medical problem.

WHAT IS HYPOTHERMIA? Normal body temperatures range from 97 to 99° F. Hypothermia is the lowering of that body core temperature due to exposure to cooler outside temperatures.

Hypothermia is divided into three classes referred to as mild, moderate and severe. Mild hypothermia is when the body temperature is 90 to 95° F. Moderate hypothermia ranges from 82 to 90° F and severe is any temperature below 82° F.

As the body temperature decreases, so do bodily functions. The metabolic functions begin to slow and eventually stop. Death will occur when hypothermia remains untreated.

HOW DOES IT OCCUR? Exposure to a cool or cold environment over a period of time will cause the body temperature to decrease. Prolonged exposure of the body without proper clothing is a leading cause for the problem. Exposure to a wet environment and wet clothing also speeds the loss of body heat.

Each year, there are about 700 deaths from hypothermia in the United States. The elderly account for over 50 percent of these deaths. With age, it becomes more difficult to regulate the body's temperature. In addition, chronic medical problems and medications may contribute to the progression of the illness. On the other end of the spectrum, small children account for the other large percentage of patients affected by hypothermia, as they are unable to tolerate prolonged exposure.

SEASONAL

WHAT ARE THE SYMPTOMS? Hypothermia occurs gradually and the first symptoms are cold hands and feet, accompanied by shivering. This may progress to a sense of feeling tired and increased confusion. Eventually, patients with more significant hypothermia will become irrational, experience loss of coordination and eventual unconsciousness. By this time, there may be very slow respirations and a very slow pulse.

HOW IS IT DIAGNOSED? Hypothermia is a clinical diagnosis based on the history of exposure and measuring the body temperature. Some standard over-the-counter thermometers do not measure temperatures below 93° F. The hospital emergency department has thermometers that are able to measure low temperatures, which is accomplished through the use of an internal body probe. Ear thermometers can be very inaccurate.

HOW IS IT TREATED? A person experiencing hypothermia needs immediate medical attention. Rapid rewarming of the body is the goal and can be started prior to the arrival of trained medical professionals. It may be necessary to call 911 for help.

Initially, it is important to get the patient into a warm environment. Movement of the patient must be done with little stimulation, as this can trigger a fatal heart arrhythmia and death. Removal of wet and cold clothing is essential.

At the hospital, several methods of rewarming are utilized including heating blankets, warm IV fluids and warm, humidified oxygen. This process can take several hours. In addition, a patient may go into cardiac arrest and CPR must be continued for a long period of time. There have been many successful resuscitations of cold water drowning victims, because the body will protect itself by slowing bodily functions and slowing the consumption of oxygen. This is called the dive reflex.

WHAT CAN I DO? As with so many medical problems, prevention is essential. Be prepared for exposure to the cooler temperatures. Wear appropriate layered clothing and be sure to cover your head. Do not drink alcoholic beverages, as they blunt the body's response to the cold weather and inhibit judgment.

Recognition of hypothermia is very important, especially when working or playing outside. Recognizing when you or a companion is suffering from the effects of the elements can be lifesaving.

In the event that you feel you are suffering from hypothermia, move into a warm environment. Drink warm fluids if possible, but never force them onto someone who seems a little confused. Hypothermia is a serious and life-threatening medical condition that can be treated. As always, seek medical attention in a timely fashion.

eczema

Each year, as we move into the cooler seasons, many people develop patches of dry, flaky and itchy skin on their hands, face, torso and other areas. There may be a variety of skin conditions that cause this, but this is most commonly caused by eczema. Eczema can exist in many different forms, so it is important to have an understanding of this condition.

WHAT IS ECZEMA? Eczema is a skin condition consisting of dry, flaky, scaling skin followed by excessive itching. In some cases, isolated patches and blisters occur. Patients affected range in age from the very young to the very old. Approximately one to two percent of all Americans have experienced eczema at some time in their life.

Eczema is more prevalent in the fall and winter months due to the cool, dry air. Eczema, a hereditary condition, may be brought on by certain foods or medicines. In addition, patients with allergies and asthma may be more likely to experience eczema. Overall, the cause of eczema is unknown.

WHAT ARE THE SYMPTOMS? Eczema is uncomfortably itchy. With the most common condition, the skin may appear red with flaking and burning. One type of eczema has small fluid filled blisters that are present on the sides of fingers and toes. The fluid within the blisters is not contagious. With time, painful cracks can also develop on the affected area.

With infants, eczema can be found on the face. In children, it may be seen in the folds of the elbows and knees. With adults, eczema may be limited to the hands, feet or torso.

HOW IS IT DIAGNOSED? Many rashes look alike, therefore eczema should be diagnosed by a health professional. Laboratory testing and a biopsy, where a skin sample is taken and looked at under a microscope, are not necessary to make the diagnosis. In complicated and confusing cases however, your doctor may choose to do a biopsy.

WHAT SHOULD I DO? Initially, a diagnosis should be made by a health care professional. After that is accomplished, several treatments are available. Skin irritants such as harsh soaps, detergents, jewelry, cosmetics and foods must be avoided. These may trigger a type of allergic reaction within the skin.

SEASONAL

The most important proactive measure that can be taken is to keep the skin appropriately moisturized. The use of skin moisturizers will keep the skin smooth and flexible, especially if used after bathing when the skin is well-hydrated. It may take some trial and error to figure out which skin conditioner is best for you.

ARE THERE PRESCRIPTION MEDICATIONS THAT HELP? It is reasonable to try some over-the-counter topical steroid creams which include one-half to one percent of hydrocortisone. This may be applied two to three times per day to the affected areas. Use should be limited, as this may cause thinning of the skin. In addition, it is important to only apply steroid cream to the extremities or the torso. Steroids should never be applied to the face or around the eyes, unless supervised by a doctor.

Based on your condition, your doctor may prescribe one of the many, stronger topical steroid creams. These steroid creams are anti-inflammatory steroids and not muscle-building or sex steroids.

WHAT CAN BE DONE TO PREVENT ECZEMA? As always, prevention is important. To prevent the onset of eczema, it's essential to take preventative steps, such as the use of moisturizers prior to the onset of cooler weather.

It is also important to avoid any foods or medications that will worsen the condition. Controlling stress may also prevent eczema.

If all of the above measures have been taken, remember to see your doctor to have the correct diagnosis made. After diagnosis, be sure to use any medications as prescribed by your doctor and continue to treat your eczema until it has completely gone away.

heat illness

For those of us in the Midwest, it seems that we wait all year for warmth and sun. When it arrives, we are not always very well prepared to deal with the short-and long-term effects of the sweltering heat. It is important that we understand how to deal with the effects of the heat of summer. All of us are at risk for the development of heat cramps, heat exhaustion and heat stroke.

WHAT HAPPENS? When the weather improves, many people gravitate to outdoor activities. But it is not only the recreational enthusiasts who are affected. Many professions involve working outside in the heat or in warm enclosures. Both of these groups of people are at risk for heat-related illnesses.

When exposed to heat for a prolonged period and the body cannot regulate heat tolerance, problems will occur. This may lead to cramping of the muscles, dehydration, weakness or significantly increased body temperature. Normal body temperature is regulated through heat production and heat loss. Heat loss usually occurs through evaporation of sweat, but when the humidity is high, this does not happen as readily.

WHAT ARE HEAT CRAMPS? After strenuous activity, muscle pain or spasm may occur. The muscles of the arms, legs and abdomen may be affected. Usually, this occurs after excessive sweating, that may cause an imbalance of the body chemicals called electrolytes.

The treatment of heat cramps involves cessation of activity and rehydration. Usually sport drinks help with rehydration and replace some of the lost electrolytes. It is important to remember that prevention is essential. Also, taking time to stretch the muscles prior to activity may help in avoiding heat cramps.

WHAT IS HEAT EXHAUSTION? When a person is exposed to a long period of high temperatures and excessive sweating occurs, heat exhaustion may result. Usually these patients are not drinking enough fluids during this time of activity and exposure. Anyone can be at risk, but the very young and the very old are at greatest risk. People with chronic medical problems and those taking a variety of medicines are also at greatest risk.

SEASONAL

When a person is experiencing heat exhaustion, they may appear pale with profuse sweating. They may complain of a headache, weakness, nausea and vomiting. The pulse may be weak and thready with a low blood pressure. This may cause a person to actually pass out. With this condition, the body temperature is normal.

The treatment involves stopping the activity in the hot environment and placing the patient in an air-conditioned room. Gradual replacement of liquids is essential. In the event that the patient is very ill and unable to tolerate these simple measures, seek medical attention.

WHAT IS HEAT STROKE? This is the most serious of all heat related illnesses. This is a true emergency and requires prompt medical attention. This condition involves the elevation of the body temperature, as the body has lost the ability to regulate temperature. The patient may appear critically ill and have a temperature of 105° F or higher. The skin will be dry and red. In the later stages of heat stroke, the patient may experience hallucinations or be unconscious.

Treatment must be provided immediately. The person needs to be removed from the hot environment and placed in an air-conditioned room. The body must be cooled through evaporation, where the body is misted with cool water and a fan is used to promote evaporation. This allows for dissipation of the heat. A person who experiences heat stroke will need to be admitted to the hospital for treatment and observation.

HOW DO I PREVENT HEAT-RELATED ILLNESS? The prevention of heat-related illness is very important. Awareness of potential exposure and preparation is very important. Be sure to wear appropriate clothing when in a hot environment. Drink fluids. Seek cool shelter and take frequent breaks from the heat. Also, there are several prescribed medications that may cause the inability to tolerate heat. Be sure to discuss this with your health care provider. Enjoy summer!

To Your Health with Dr. Wojo

rhinitis

With the onset of spring and the return of vegetation, there is also a return of runny noses, sneezing, itching and red eyes. Many people love the weather, but hate the development of their seasonal allergies!

Seasonal allergies, also called seasonal rhinitis, affect up to 30 million Americans and it is in the top ten chronic medical conditions, out-ranking heart disease. About 1.5 million school days and 3.5 million workdays are missed due to this acute and chronic medical condition.

WHAT IS SEASONAL RHINITIS? Seasonal rhinitis is the irritation of the nasal mucosa or inner surfaces, due to allergens. These allergens may come from pollen, dust or molds. When inhaled onto the nasal surface, an allergic response begins. A whole cascade of events occurs within the body, that may be manifested by a variety of symptoms.

WHAT ARE THE SYMPTOMS? Seasonal rhinitis may present with a stuffy or runny nose with clear discharge. There may be some associated congestion, itching, sneezing and red eyes. The symptoms are somewhat progressive in nature. The symptoms are usually not life-threatening and may resolve within a few days.

WHO IS AFFECTED? A patient of any age may be affected by seasonal allergies. The most common patients are children and adolescents. It is unusual to develop this at a very late age, unless the patient has a previous history of this condition. Therefore, the allergy condition may be quiet for a number of years and then it may re-present itself. If allergies are developed in the twenties, they will usually stick with the patient throughout the remainder of their lifetime.

Factors that affect the development include heredity. It is known that if both parents have seasonal allergies, there is a 75 percent chance that their child will be affected. With only one parent being affected, that risk drops to 50 percent. But, heredity is not necessary to develop these allergies.

HOW IS IT DIAGNOSED? As with so many conditions, it is important for your health care provider to obtain a very comprehensive history of the disease process. Things to be considered would include the timetable of the symptoms, types of symptoms, known irritants, family history and factors that may improve the condition.

SEASONAL

Initially, whether seen in your doctor's office or in the emergency department, a great deal of testing is not required. Based on the history and presentation, a plan of treatment will be outlined. Eventually, a referral to an allergy specialist may be warranted. A patient needs to be off their allergy medicines for a couple of weeks, prior to allergy testing. The most common tests include skin patch testing, in order to define offending allergens.

WHAT IS THE TREATMENT? Over the past 50 years, the mainstay of treatment has included the use of antihistamines. There are over 100 antihistamines on the market in both prescribed and over-the-counter forms. Each has its merit.

The first generation antihistamines have proven efficacy and are inexpensive. Most are over-the-counter. Unfortunately, they cause drowsiness. This is the most common side effect. Of interest, most over-the-counter sleep aids are these same antihistamines.

The second-generation antihistamines have gained widespread usage and are quite successful at treating allergic rhinitis. They must be prescribed by your health care provider, are costly, and usually do not cause drowsiness. Other side effects are minimal.

Other medications may be used including nasal inhalants, steroids and eye drops. The simple goal of therapy is "to get the red out"! For chronic conditions, your doctor may choose to initiate immunotherapy, commonly referred to as allergy shots.

WHAT SHOULD I DO? As with all medical conditions, it is essential to have the proper diagnosis made. The offending allergens must be defined and avoided if possible. During peak allergy seasons, a course of prevention may be considered. This may include the use of over-the-counter and prescribed antihistamines. Your health care provider may choose to add some additional medications or institute a series of allergy shots.

In the event that you experience severe distress including shortness of breath, throat swelling or itching, or a significant rash, you must see your doctor immediately. This may include a trip to the emergency department. It is always important to seek help when you have questions, as this condition is fully treatable, making life more tolerable.

seasonal
allergies

The spring season is one of my favorite times of the year. The sun is usually shining, the grass is starting to green up and trees are sprouting their leaves. Unfortunately, at this time of the year, the air is filled with pollen and allergens. While enjoying the outdoors, I am sneezing, my eyes are watering and my nose is congested. Sound familiar? I also hear that each year is the worst for allergies. I think that we just forget how miserable we felt last year.

WHAT ARE SEASONAL ALLERGIES? An allergic response occurs when our bodies activate our immune system to respond to common everyday substances. This response may be caused by a genetic factor or an environmental factor.

During spring, the air is filled with pollens from trees and plants. As this vegetation begins to bloom, pollen is released and it may affect some humans and animals. The mission of the pollen is to fertilize other parts of the plant, but it usually gets into our nose instead! Depending on the region and climate, one can usually expect to experience symptoms during the same time every year. The responsible culprits include birch trees, maples, oaks, flowering trees and grasses.

This is a fairly common problem in the United States with 35 million people suffering from seasonal allergies. Of this number, about 5 million are children.

WHAT ARE THE SYMPTOMS? It may be hard to distinguish the difference between a cold and allergies. But, in spring, the symptoms are probably due to allergies. A person may experience sneezing, a runny nose, itching eyes, congestion, coughing, and a headache. Usually, there will not be a fever, unlike with a viral respiratory illness.

For some people with underlying medical problems like asthma, allergies may worsen their condition. Asthmatics may have a tough time breathing and may require more medications than usual.

CAN ALLERGIES BE PREVENTED? Though they cannot be prevented, the severity of the attack can be minimized. When one knows that they are susceptible to this condition, avoidance is essential. Simple measures include keeping the house closed up and running the air-conditioning if necessary. Granted, the fresh air after a long winter is appealing, but it may make life miserable.

It helps to stay indoors on windy days, as the pollen is being blown around and driven onto our bodies. Dehumidifying the air in the house is helpful as well. High-efficiency particulate air filters do work and are quite effective in keeping the house allergen free. With more severe cases, individuals may have to aggressively clean their homes, including the bedding. Beds may need to be enclosed with allergy covers. All of these measures may make spring a little more bearable.

WHAT IS THE TREATMENT? Medical therapy may involve several approaches. For the less severe cases, over-the-counter allergy medications are quite effective. These medicines may include Benadryl, Chlor-Trimeton or Tavist. Other medications that are now over-the-counter include Claritin, which is a non-sedating antihistamine.

With more severe cases, prescription medications must be used including a variety of other non-sedating histamines and oral steroids like prednisone. Some people may require the use of oral decongestants or nasal sprays. Nasal sprays include a pure decongestant or a nasal steroid. This helps in calming the inflammatory response.

Lastly, a visit to an allergist may be in order. Patch testing may specifically identify offending substances. With very severe cases, allergy desensitization shots may help alleviate the problem. This can be a fairly long, drawn-out process, so this issue must be addressed with your primary care provider.

Spring is a great time of the year, but we can be slowed down by this simple problem. Usually, the condition is not life-threatening, so a trip to your local drug store may help in lessening the symptoms. Your pharmacist may point you in the right direction for some cost-effective treatment.

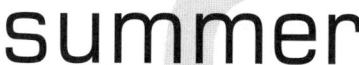

summer

In summer, everyone seems to be outside enjoying the nice weather. Outdoor activity has increased by about a hundred fold and the young and old are participating in a variety of things that can't be done in December. It is essential to not spoil these times of travel and fun with a visit to the emergency department (ED). Historically, ED visits increase in number during the summer months. These visits range from generalized illness to trauma.

WHAT ARE COMMON EMERGENCY DEPARTMENT VISITS? As the United States population continues to age, a large percentage of patients that visit the ED are the elderly. Nationally, in the past 10 years, ED volumes have increased by 20 percent. Total ED visits have grown from 92 million patient encounters to 108 million patient encounters. This is not unique to any particular geographic region, but it is a national trend.

Many elderly people are burdened with chronic medical problems such as coronary artery disease, congestive heart failure, high blood pressure, high cholesterol, diabetes and emphysema. All of these conditions contribute to a state that mandates a visit to the emergency department and possibly hospital admission.

Warm, humid weather seems to worsen respiratory illness and patients with emphysema require acute medical care. Many times, prolonged hot weather contributes to heat-related illness that weakens a frail body. Immediate intervention may be necessary to rapidly cool the patient and replenish lost body electrolytes.

Even though it seems that diseases of the elderly are chronic and need attention year round, the summer months seem to worsen some of those conditions. Overall, a large percentage of the practice of emergency medicine has focused on treating the elderly.

WHAT ARE COMMON SUMMER VISITS? The summer months encourage outdoor sporting activities and the incidence of minor orthopedic trauma seems to increase. This may include a variety of sprains, strains, fractures and lacerations. It is really important to understand your physical limitations prior to participating in some activities.

SEASONAL

For example, if you are not an avid water-skier, be sure to know your limitations. It is essential to wear appropriate personal flotation devices and know the area where you are skiing. Be sure not to mix excessive alcohol with boating, as it is dangerous and against the law!

Outdoor cooking is always fun, but not without danger. Be sure to understand your grilling devices and do not take chances with malfunctions. NEVER start a fire using gasoline. Many family gatherings have been spoiled by thoughtless acts that require a prolonged stay at a burn center. It is important that if burned, remove the patient from further danger, activate 911, rapidly cool the burn, do not apply ointments, and seek medical attention.

ARE THERE OTHER PREVENTABLE INJURIES IN THE SUMMER? Yes. The most common serious injury that could have been minor, through the use of a helmet, is a head injury. Each year, numerous injuries to the head require intensive medical care, prolonged hospitalization, rehabilitation, and unfortunately can lead to permanent damage. A large percentage of these cases could have been prevented through the use of a helmet.

It should be a mandate with all children and minors that a helmet be worn when bicycling, scootering, skate boarding and roller blading. Hard surfaces can cause bruising and bleeding in the brain, that if left untreated, will lead to death. Surprisingly, a great deal of force is not always required to cause a severe injury to the head. The elderly have a greater likelihood of severe brain injury with a blow to the head, as do young children.

SWIMMING. Some of the most tragic accidents that we see each summer are associated with water sports and swimming. Most drownings are preventable. Be sure to supervise your children when they are swimming. No one should ever swim alone in a lake or river. Be sure to know where the currents are, and swim in appropriately designated areas.

When diving into a pool or lake, know the depth. Cervical spine injuries associated with diving accidents are almost always associated with permanent paralysis. Many of these injuries are related to alcohol. A foolish choice may result in quadriplegia and a lifetime of disability.

This is a great time of year in the north, so enjoy it. A little bit of preparation and common sense will keep you injury free. Be sure to condition yourself for new physical activities and do not take any shortcuts on safety. Alcohol in excess will usually cut short many of these activities, with long-term sequelae. Follow these simple tips and have a great summer season!

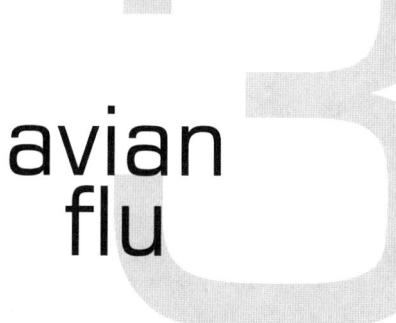

avian flu

There is certainly some concern in Asian countries regarding avian influenza that is infecting the bird population and humans. There are no documented cases of avian influenza in the United States, but precautionary measures are in place for those that travel to Asian countries. This is primarily a disease of domestic poultry and the deaths have been incidental to contact with the infected birds. In Hong Kong, this human disease killed nearly a million chickens.

WHAT IS AVIAN INFLUENZA? Avian influenza is a virus that infects mostly domestic poultry and some pigs. The viral illness has two forms. The first is a mild form that causes minimal symptoms in birds such as ruffled feathers and decreased egg production.

In the severe form, called highly pathogenic avian influenza, the onset is very sudden and death occurs in 100 percent of all birds. Once infected, a bird will die within 24 hours of the onset of the infection. Among birds, the virus is very contagious. Avian influenza does not directly infect humans.

Avian influenza is a subtype of influenza that is very similar to Influenza A, which causes upper respiratory illness and pneumonia in humans. It is important to remember that the bird flu only infects domesticated birds, and usually not birds in the wild.

HOW ARE THESE BIRDS INFECTED? The domesticated birds such as chickens, ducks and turkeys are raised in close quarters. When a certain bird is infected, it acts as a host for the virus that is carried in the intestines of the bird. The virus is then shed in the saliva, nasal secretions and feces.

Other birds that have contact with these secretions become infected. Most of the viruses only cause mild symptoms, but the more serious strain of the virus will cause death of the bird. There are a variety of subtypes with the most aggressive being identified as strains H5 and H7.

ARE HUMANS INFECTED? Yes, but rarely. The documented cases of human infections have been confined mostly to Asian countries. Currently, the most aggressive strain is H5N1 and caution must be exercised when found in the poultry population.

VIRAL

The cases of human infection were found in individuals who had been in close contact with the birds. Several individuals who were infected did recover from the severe respiratory illness. It is important to note that there has been limited documentation of cases of human-to-human transmission of the virus.

WHAT ARE THE SYMPTOMS OF THE INFECTION IN HU-MANS? Avian influenza presents with symptoms similar to that of Influenza A. It is primarily a respiratory illness where a patient may experience a sore throat, fever, cough and muscle aches. More severe causes may lead to pneumonia, respiratory distress and failure, as well as death.

WHAT IS THE TREATMENT? Just like with Influenza A, Avian Influenza responds to the same anti-viral medications that are used in the United States such as amantadine, rimantadine and zanamivir. These anti-viral medications have been prescribed to millions of people in the United States for the treatment of Influenza A and in order to prevent it. In addition, humans infected with the virus must be given supportive treatment, which may involve rehydration, respiratory support and hospitalization.

CAN THIS DISEASE SPREAD? There is always the possibility for the spread of disease outside of Asia. The World Health Organization and the Centers for Disease Control are monitoring the situation very closely. International trade of poultry is limited and travelers are being monitored. Travelers to the endemic areas are encouraged to stay away from open poultry markets, but other significant restrictions are not required.

Very close surveillance of the disease patterns is occurring and research centers around the change of the virus into a more aggressive strain. The situation is under control and at the present time, there is little worry of a severe outbreak of the bird flu in the United States.

bronchitis

Do you have a cold? A persistent cough? Fever? Pain in your chest when you cough? You may be experiencing a bout of bronchitis.

WHAT IS BRONCHITIS? Bronchitis is an inflammation of the bronchial or breathing tubes that allow passage of air into the lungs. These air passages become inflamed when exposed to irritants such as smoke, pollutants, viruses or bacteria. The cells lining the bronchioles become irritated and swollen, eventually producing a large amount of mucous that constitutes phlegm.

ARE THERE DIFFERENT TYPES OF BRONCHITIS? Yes. A person may experience an acute form of bronchitis, that is secondary to a new irritant such as a virus. A majority of cases of bronchitis are caused by viruses and will usually resolve on their own.

Patients with underlying lung disease, such as emphysema, may experience chronic bronchitis. This involves excessive mucous production which may last from three months to multiple years. Many times, there may be difficulty in coughing up the phlegm.

On the surface of the bronchioles are cilia that are little brushes. These brushes beat rhythmically, removing irritants. When infected or damaged by smoke, the cilia do not work as effectively, contributing to chronic respiratory infections.

WHAT ARE THE SYMPTOMS? In general, bronchitis usually starts as a cold or upper respiratory infection. The virus that causes the cold settles into the bronchioles where they become swollen and begin producing more phlegm.

With this increased mucous production, a cough will develop. Prolonged coughing may be part of bronchitis. A patient may feel short of breath and develop some pain in the chest secondary to the coughing. Other symptoms of the viral syndrome may include wheezing, fever, chills and aches.

HOW IS IT DIAGNOSED? Bronchitis is a clinical diagnosis made by your health care provider, who may choose to do some testing. This testing may be laboratory analysis of the phlegm including culture. Blood tests may be ordered to check for other serious problems. With significant shortness of breath and chest pain, a chest x-ray may be ordered to primarily rule out pneumonia.

VIRAL

Usually, young healthy people with no underlying medical conditions require no testing. Patients with more serious health problems may require laboratory and x-ray analysis to further assess the status of the situation.

HOW IS IT TREATED? Bronchitis may be treated symptomatically with over-the-counter cold medications. With more advanced cases and wheezing, asthma medications such as inhalers may help. These must be prescribed by your doctor.

It is important to determine if the cause of bronchitis is secondary to bacteria. If it is, an antibiotic will be prescribed. It is very important to remember that viruses cause the majority of bronchitis cases and antibiotics should not be taken. The overuse of antibiotics has become an international health care issue that requires close surveillance. The over-prescribing of antibiotics has caused a significant problem of resistance, whereby simple bacterial infections now require expensive, high-powered antibiotics.

WHAT CAN I DO? Prevention is key. Smoking contributes to 90 percent of chronic cases and therefore, stopping this habit is essential.

The spread of the virus occurs through respiratory droplets released by coughing and sneezing. Good hand washing helps with preventing the spread of the viruses. Also, staying out of smoky and polluted environments can be a great preventative measure. If you are infected, avoid close personal contact for 24 to 48 hours.

WHEN SHOULD I SEE THE DOCTOR? In the event that you begin to experience severe shortness of breath and cough, it is reasonable to be evaluated by your health care provider. Also, having a persistent cough of one month's duration merits a visit to the doctor's office to rule out any other serious problems.

Overall, it is important to remember that bronchitis is a fairly common health problem during the winter months. All cases of bronchitis do not require the use of antibiotics and be sure not to pressure your doctor into prescribing one when they are not indicated. In conclusion, bronchitis can be a self-limited disease that may take a few weeks to resolve. In the event that you feel that your condition is deteriorating or you are severely short of breath, you need to seek medical attention.

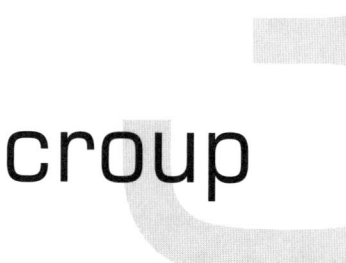

croup

There is nothing more terrifying than waking up at 2:00 a.m. to your child's barking, seal-like cough and realizing they are having trouble breathing. What they may be experiencing is actually croup and luckily there is a way you can treat it without a visit to the hospital.

WHAT IS CROUP? Croup is a viral infection that affects the upper airway of children ages six months to six years. It is caused by one of several types of respiratory viruses invading the nose and throat. The child's airway, from the voice box to the bronchioles, will become infected. Once this happens, there will be swelling and narrowing of the air passages and mucous production, resulting in small, constricted airways. The sound associated with such an infection ranges from a high-pitched barking cough to severe respiratory distress.

HOW DOES THIS HAPPEN? During the late fall and winter months, a child will be exposed to several respiratory viruses. These viruses are passed from person to person by general contact. They often settle in the nose and throat and begin to grow from there. It will take a couple of days for this to happen, but once it happens, the child is at risk for inflammation of the airways. The symptoms of croup may last for a couple of days.

WHO IS AFFECTED? In general, due to their smaller airways, young children are at higher risk to become infected and develop croup. Young boys more frequently sufferer from croup by a ratio of 2:1. Due to the increased size of the airways, it is rare to see children, boys or girls, older than the age of eight who experience croup.

WHAT ARE THE SYMPTOMS? As noted, a bout of croup usually happens in the middle of the night. In addition to the cough, a child may also have symptoms of a respiratory illness with a low-grade fever, runny nose and sore throat. The cough of croup sounds just like a barking seal. It is high-pitched and almost deafening. You may also see some flaring of the child's nostrils and sinking of the chest with breathing. This is called retraction.

WHAT SHOULD I DO? When you go to the aid of your child, you must be supportive. When convinced that they are experiencing croup, you can do several things. If they are experiencing severe respiratory distress, you must call 911. If the condition is mild, a few home remedies have been proven helpful throughout the years.

VIRAL

First, start a hot shower and allow the bathroom to steam up. Be sure the exhaust fan is not on. This will usually take about five minutes. While you are waiting, reassure your child. You may want to take them out into the cool nighttime air. This calms the airway.

After the bathroom is adequately humidified, take your child into the steamy room and allow them to sit there for up to 30 minutes. This may be enough to calm the airways and thin the mucous secretions. It this is not working, a visit to the emergency department is necessary.

WHAT CAN I EXPECT AT THE HOSPITAL? Once the diagnosis of croup is confirmed, a breathing treatment of humidified adrenalin (epinephrine) is given. This will be followed by a single dose of an oral steroid. These are all safe medications and widely used.

There are times when a child may have thick, infected secretions. It may be necessary that they take an antibiotic, but this is infrequent. Remember, croup is a viral infection and does not require antibiotics. After a period of observation, you may be sent home.

CAN CROUP BE PREVENTED? No. There are no vaccines to prevent the spread of the respiratory viruses. It is important to be aware that when your child has a viral upper respiratory infection they may be at risk for croup. You need to be prepared in order to deal with the situation. In general, croup is not life-threatening, but it is a serious respiratory illness that requires prompt attention. If there is any question of the severity of the illness or the cause, always seek professional medical attention.

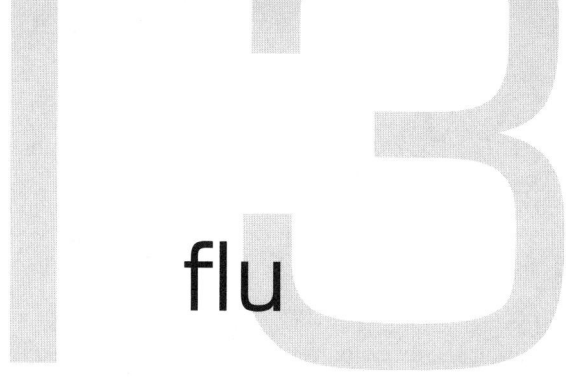

flu

Usually after the holidays, a viral respiratory illness begins to present itself. Doctors' offices, clinics and hospitals become inundated with patients seeking a cure for this problem. The epidemic usually lasts about a month and is very contagious, but usually not life threatening. The diagnosis: Influenza.

WHAT IS INFLUENZA? Influenza is a viral respiratory illness that usually presents during the winter months. Each year, a different strain of virus invades the body and different vaccines are made to prevent development of the disease process. Most often Influenza A and less often Influenza B, are diagnosed. The virus, commonly referred to as the flu, invades the respiratory passages of the body.

HOW DOES IT DEVELOP? Once the respiratory virus becomes prevalent, it is passed in respiratory droplets from person to person by direct contact or indirect contact such as coughing and sneezing. Once a person is infected, the virus invades the respiratory passages of the body. The onset of symptoms begins within a day and may last up to a week.

WHAT ARE THE SYMPTOMS? The progression of symptoms is generally quite rapid. A person will have a sudden onset of fever, dry cough, sore throat, runny nose, and generalized aches and pains. It is not unusual to see fevers as high as 105° F. Patients complain that they feel as if they have been run over by a truck! Usually, influenza does not have gastrointestinal symptoms such as vomiting and diarrhea.

HOW IS IT DIAGNOSED? During the initial phase of community epidemics, health care providers must be suspect for the presence of influenza. Laboratory testing will include a nasal swab that will check for the presence of the influenza virus.

As the community epidemic progresses, health care providers can make the diagnosis on the basis of history and physical exam. Patients that are in poor health are at greater risk for complications and may therefore mandate further blood testing and x-rays. Usually, minimal workup is necessary in healthy people.

VIRAL

WHAT SHOULD I DO? As with so many medical conditions, prevention is essential. Each fall, the current influenza vaccination is available and should be considered. People with chronic underlying medical conditions should always be vaccinated, as should health workers and patients over the age of 50. People with an allergy to eggs cannot be vaccinated.

In the event that you become ill, the treatment is symptomatic. This involves rest, fluid hydration and fever control with acetaminophen and ibuprofen. There are a variety of medications that can be prescribed by your health care providers that can shorten the course of the disease process. These medicines are only effective if prescribed within the first 24 to 48 hours of the disease course.

WHEN SHOULD I SEEK MEDICAL ATTENTION? In general, young healthy patients will not experience any significant problem in combatting the three-to-five-day course of the illness. Those at major risk for flu complications include the very young and patients over the age of 65. Dehydration is a major risk factor in the younger population.

In the older patient population, the major risk factor is the development of pneumonia, that may be bacterial in nature. This may require a course of antibiotics as well as the use of an antiviral medication. It is important to note that antibiotics do not treat influenza, but they may be used to treat a complication as a result of the viral illness. Many elderly patients may require hospitalization for close management and follow up of their primary disease and complications. As always, in the event that you have any questions or concerns about your illness, seek expert advice from your primary health care provider.

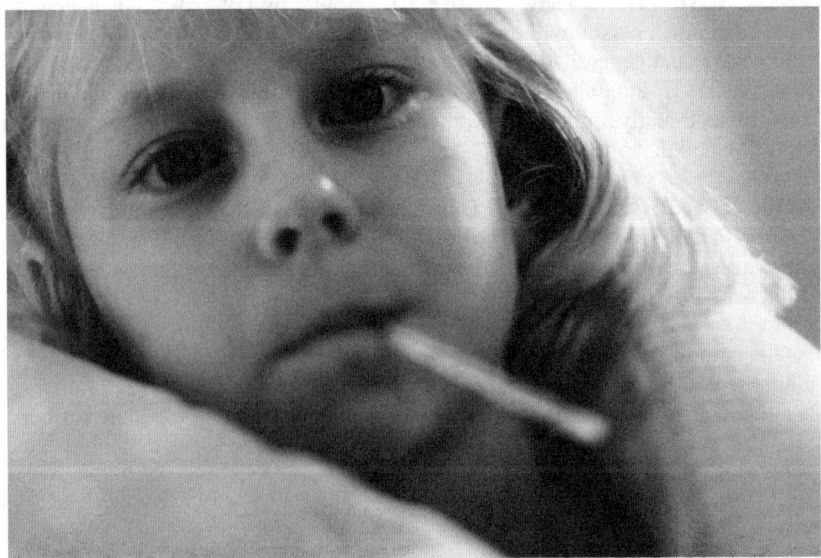

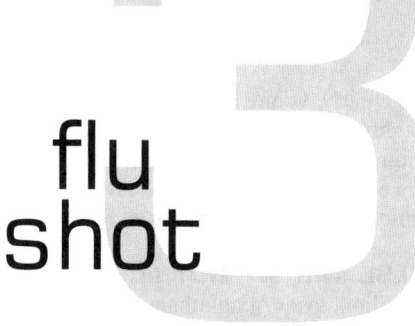

flu shot

As we move into the winter months, it is time to protect ourselves against influenza (flu). Whenever an announcement is made that there is going to be a shortage of influenza vaccinations in the United States, a wave of panic rises throughout the country. Is there a reason to panic? Probably not.

WHY ARE THERE SHORTAGES? There are two major producers of influenza or flu vaccine in the world. Aventis produces and distributes about 55 million doses of flu vaccine in the United States and Chiron, a British company, distributes about 46 million doses. At times, vaccines have been found to be contaminated and thus production is shut down and doses of flu vaccine are destroyed.

The manufacture of the vaccine involves the growing of the virus in eggs and takes several months to accomplish. The virus is then killed and the inactivated vaccine is injected into a patient. Since the whole process takes a considerable amount of time, it is impossible for manufacturers to begin immediate production of additional vaccines. Since this process is somewhat old-fashioned, companies are looking at other ways to develop and distribute flu vaccines in the near future.

WHAT SHOULD WE DO? The Centers for Disease Control (CDC) immediately responds to the the shortage of vaccines—which is not deemed a catastrophe. Guidelines for the distribution of the limited supply are made by the CDC.

People at risk for being infected with the flu and those who cannot withstand this insult are advised to be vaccinated. For example, health care workers should be immunized since they are in close contact with patients infected by the flu.

Other people who should be vaccinated are the older population, ages 65 and above. With aging, it is a little harder to fight off this respiratory illness. Patients in nursing homes should be vaccinated, because the disease can spread rapidly throughout a facility, causing serious illness in already debilitated patients.

VIRAL

Besides the elderly, young children ages 6-23 months may have a more difficult time fighting off the flu, so they should be immunized. Others that should consider immunization are those people with chronic medical problems, who would have a difficult time fighting and recovering from the flu. The CDC has set forth guidelines that can be viewed at www.cdc.gov.

WHAT ELSE CAN WE DO? In addition to the standard flu shot, there are about 1.1 million doses of an inhaled flu vaccine. This is made by a different process and involves the inhalation of a weaker form of a live flu virus. This exposure allows a person to develop immunity through this exposure. This is a fairly effective preventative measure.

For the healthy person, there are several things that can be done to diminish your chances of getting the flu. This involves good hand washing and decreasing your chances of exposure. In addition to that, if you are infected with the flu, the illness is self-limited. Fluids and fever control are essential. Usually, there are no complications, but you may be set back and out of work for a few days.

Another method of prevention may involve the administration of several different oral medications that can either prevent the development of the infection once exposed or shorten the course. Those medications are amantadine, rimantadine, zanamivir, or oseltamivir. These medicines are fairly safe and quite effective. They range in price from inexpensive to fairly expensive.

Lastly, it is important to discuss this health maintenance issue with your health care provider who can help determine whether you are at risk for the development of the flu and more serious complications. Options for treatment will be provided. Remember, this is not a major crisis, so do not panic. If you are an at-risk individual, appropriate treatment will be provided.

hand-foot-and-mouth disease

Each year, as the summer comes to a close and fall begins, many children become ill with a number of symptoms that include a fever, mouth ulcers or blisters on the hands and feet. This is a fairly benign, but painful condition, that is called Hand-Foot-and-Mouth Disease (HFMD). For once, a medical term that can easily be remembered!

WHAT IS HFMD? HFMD is an acute viral illness that presents itself with a fairly high fever, fatigue, sore throat and blisters on the hands and feet. The mouth will have canker sores on the gums, inside cheeks and the tonsils. These sores may appear pale with a yellow base. The blisters on the hands and feet are usually on the sides of the fingers and toes and are small with clear fluid. It is also possible that the genitalia can be affected.

HOW DO YOU GET HFMD? This disease is spread from person to person by direct contact with nasal and oral secretions. Small droplets also can be spread through sneezing and coughing. These viral droplets either get on the skin or the oral surfaces and eventually invade the body. HFMD is very contagious and can easily be spread through facilities such as daycare centers.

WHO GETS HFMD? In general, children up to the age of 10 are most frequently affected. The distribution is the same among boys and girls, but it seems that boys' symptoms are more severe. It is not unusual for adults to be infected as well. This is especially common when a parent's children are sick. Many times, adults will only have a part of the clinical syndrome, such as a sore throat or blisters.

WHAT CAN I EXPECT? Once exposed, a child may feel a little ill before the entire syndrome manifests itself. After being exposed, it may take up to a week for the full condition to be present. The incubation period is listed as three to six days. Once the child is sick, the condition may last for about three to four days, with complete resolution within a week.

WHAT SHOULD I DO? Initially, it is important to make the proper diagnosis. After this is made, there is no formal treatment or cure. The syndrome must run its course.

VIRAL

It is important to treat the fever with acetaminophen (Tylenol) and ibuprofen (Advil, Motrin). Remember to avoid the use of plain aspirin in children! Aspirin and a viral illness are a bad mix and can cause a life-threatening condition called Reye's syndrome.

Children with HFMD can become dehydrated because a sore throat makes it difficult to swallow. Keep the Popsicles and fluids at hand. Rarely, children need to be admitted to the hospital when infected with HFMD.

Another home remedy that may ease the pain of the sore throat is equal parts of Benadryl suspension and Maalox. Benadryl has some anesthetic qualities that numb the throat. In addition, Maalox had some sedating properties. A swish and swallow mixture may be recommended by your doctor.

CAN THIS BE PREVENTED? As with most respiratory illnesses, good hygiene and hand washing are essential. There are no vaccines that can prevent this infection. In addition, it is important to keep your child out of daycare when they are infected until their condition has begun to improve. The fluid in the blisters is not contagious, but it should be avoided.

It is important to make the correct diagnosis initially. Your doctor is usually aware when there seems to be an outbreak in the community. It is rare when epidemics are present. Supportive treatment is essential and complications are infrequent. Most importantly, when you have questions or concerns, see your primary health care provider.

hepatitis A virus (HAV)

In 2003, The Center for Disease Control documented 25 cases of Hepatitis A in nine states, including Wisconsin. Many of the infected victims had visited an outdoor music concert that involved large crowds with poor sanitation and camping facilities.

WHAT IS HEPATITIS A? Hepatitis A is a viral infection that affects the liver. The liver will become inflamed, painful and swollen. Hepatitis simply means an inflammation or infection of the liver. Additionally, there are several different viruses such as B, C, D and E, which also inflame the liver, but each virus has specific characteristics, signs and symptoms.

Hepatitis A is specifically an RNA virus that is related to poor sanitation and is passed on from person to person. This is one of the most common forms of acute viral hepatitis in the world. In the United States, there are approximately 138,000 cases diagnosed each year. Ten years ago, there were less than 100 documented deaths annually from Hepatitis A.

HOW DOES IT OCCUR? The Hepatitis A virus comes from infected stool and is passed from human to human. The passage of the virus can occur due to poor hand washing, poor sanitation, food handled by an infected person, sewer-contaminated water or eating shellfish caught in contaminated waters. Many unsuspecting Americans have been infected from shellfish over the years.

WHAT ARE THE SIGNS AND SYMPTOMS? It may take from four to six weeks after exposure for any symptoms to occur. Cases can be mild with no change in health or obvious symptoms. Other cases may be much more serious.

VIRAL

In general, flu-like symptoms may eventually develop. These symptoms are very nonspecific including loss of appetite, nausea, vomiting, fever, generalized aches and fatigue. As the disease progresses, a patient may notice dark colored urine, which is secondary to an elevation in a liver and blood by-product called bilirubin.

Bilirubin is a dark-pigmented chemical that contributes to jaundice. As Hepatitis A progresses, a patient may develop a yellow color to the skin and whites of the eyes. Jaundice is a marker for a serious medical condition and must be evaluated by a health care provider immediately when it is detected.

HOW IS HEPATITIS A DIAGNOSED? The diagnosis of Hepatitis A is made through obtaining a thorough history of travel events and exposure, especially in the two months prior to the evaluation. A physical examination may reveal pain over the liver, which is in the upper right quadrant of the abdomen. The skin will be checked for jaundice and blood work will be obtained. The blood work may reveal an elevation in the liver enzymes, and specific antibodies can be checked for the presence of Hepatitis A.

HOW IS IT TREATED? There is no specific treatment for Hepatitis A. All treatment is generally supportive. Some patients may require hospitalization for rehydration and intravenous therapy. It is important to avoid any liver irritants such as alcohol and acetaminophen (Tylenol) for six months. Foods should be high in protein and eaten in small amounts due to the presence of nausea. Keeping hydrated with fluids is important.

WHAT ELSE CAN I DO? Prevention is essential! Avoid close contact with infected individuals and high-risk environments. Be sure to wash your hands frequently.

Hepatitis A vaccinations are very effective. The immunization consists of two shots six months apart. The shots are recommended when traveling to underdeveloped countries, and for homosexual males, illegal drug users who inject drugs, and those with chronic medical problems such as liver disease.

As always, if you have a concern about this medical condition, seek advice from your health care provider. You may be able to prevent an avoidable illness, but if infected, your chances of recovery are good.

monkeypox

DO YOU NEED TO WORRY ABOUT BUYING A PET? Probably not. After the outbreak of monkeypox virus in Wisconsin, Illinois and Indiana, the Center for Disease Control (CDC) and State and local health authorities swiftly identified the problem and took action to stop the spread of the disease.

WHAT IS THE MONKEYPOX VIRUS? This virus is from a class of orthopoxviruses that were initially discovered in African monkeys in the 1950s. Later studies showed that the virus infected ground squirrels, rats, mice and rabbits. Viruses that are similar in nature included smallpox and cowpox.

It was not until 1970, when a smallpox-type illness was identified in humans in Africa. The first reported cases of human infection by monkeypox occurred the first week of June 2003 in the United States.

WHAT ARE SIGNS AND SYMPTOMS? Humans that are infected with the monkeypox virus must first be exposed to an infected animal. Within two weeks of the exposure to an infected animal, a patient may complain of a variety of vague viral-illness type symptoms.

The symptoms have included fever, chills, generalized aches, sweats and a dry cough. Within one to ten days, a rash will develop. The rash will initially be flat and red. It will then blister, appear infected with pus and crust over. Some of the lesions may develop into skin ulcers.

HOW IS THE VIRUS TRANSMITTED? The cases in the Midwest were all related to infected prairie dogs from one particular distributor in Illinois. It appears that the prairie dogs were initially exposed to an infected Gambian giant rat that was imported from Africa. The giant rat was the carrier of the monkeypox virus and it infected the prairie dogs through close contact. The prairie dogs were sold in Wisconsin, Illinois and Indiana.

Humans became infected through close contact with their new pet, the prairie dog. It is thought that the virus is spread via respiratory droplets and close face-to-face contact. Additionally, infected body fluids may contain the virus and cause the spread of the illness. It is possible that humans may transmit the illness to one another by close contact.

WHAT IS THE TREATMENT? There is no specific treatment for the viral illness associated with exposure to the monkeypox virus. Patients are treated supportively, which has included isolation and hospitalization. The chance of death is fairly remote in humans, but some of the infected animals have died.

It was interesting to note that the CDC released the use of the smallpox vaccine as a preventative treatment. This vaccine is effective in preventing the development of the viral illness in exposed patients up to 85 percent of the time. The vaccine is being made available to people exposed to infected animals, health care workers and veterinary workers. The vaccine should be given within two weeks of exposure to an infected animal.

ARE THERE OTHER RECOMMENDATIONS? The CDC has released some home management guidelines for infected patients that do not require hospitalization. This includes 21 days of home isolation, use of respiratory masks by family members, good hygiene and hand washing, standard laundry procedures, normal dishwashing procedures and the use of household disinfectants.

DO I NEED TO WORRY? Probably not! It is important to contact your veterinarian if you have concerns about your animal, prior to transporting it to their office. Provisions must be made so that other animals are not infected through the transport process. Additionally, if you have personal health care concerns, contact your primary health care provider.

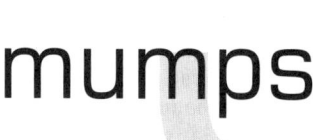

mumps

I have been practicing medicine for 16 years and have never seen a case of the mumps. It is interesting to note, that growing up in the 1960s and early 1970s, I remember hearing of cases in our area. Since that time, the disease has almost been nonexistent, with the exception of a couple outbreaks in the 1980s. This attests to the importance of childhood immunizations.

WHAT IS MUMPS? Mumps is a systemic viral illness caused by a Rubulavirus. The most common physical complaint is swelling of the parotid gland, a salivary gland that is located just in front of the ear. When this occurs, the patient looks like a chipmunk that is storing nuts in their cheeks, preparing for the winter.

WHAT ARE THE SYMPTOMS? This is a self-limited disease that may last seven to ten days. A patient with mumps will present with swelling and pain in the parotid gland. It may take two to three weeks to develop the illness after exposure. There may be increased pain with chewing and there may also be a fever. Other symptoms can include a headache, generalized aches and pains and a loss of appetite. The symptoms are usually more pronounced in adults as opposed to children.

The biggest concern with mumps is potential complications in teenaged and adult patients. In the male patient, there is risk for infection in the testicles. Usually, only one testicle is involved, but it may shrink in size after the infection. In more rare cases, both testicles become involved. This leads to a high rate of sterility. Fortunately, studies have shown that there is no increase in testicular cancer after a bout of mumps.

Just like with any viral illness, other complications include meningitis and encephalitis. Meningitis involves infection of the cerebral spinal fluid in the spinal column and encephalitis is an infection of the brain. The most prevalent symptom is a headache. The patient may be very uncomfortable while infected, but almost everyone fully recovers with no problems. It is rare to suffer long-term complications after meningitis or encephalitis caused by the mumps virus.

VIRAL

HOW IS THIS DIAGNOSED? Mumps is a clinical diagnosis whereby the examination of the patient will usually lead to the correct diagnosis. Laboratory confirmation is not necessary. But during an outbreak it may be essential to determine the incidence of the spread of the disease. A variety of lab tests are able to confirm the presence of the mumps virus and the body's immune response. The virus may be isolated from blood, urine or cerebral spinal fluid.

HOW DOES THIS SPREAD? Mumps is only found in humans, who act as the host. The virus is spread through respiratory droplets from coughing or sneezing. It is highly contagious and that is why we see epidemics in populations that live in close quarters such as on college campuses or in the military.

WHAT IS THE TREATMENT? As with any viral illness, the treatment is supportive. This involves fever control with acetaminophen and ibuprofen. It is important to prevent the spread of the disease, as it is highly contagious.

Most importantly, prevention is essential. The mumps vaccine, which is part of the series of shots given to children, must be given first at around age one with a second dose around age four. This is part of the MMR vaccine, which stands for measles-mumps-rubella. The vaccine is quite effective, leading to about 95 percent immunity.

Mumps is a significant health problem in certain areas. In the event that you are concerned that you have been exposed or have become infected, you should seek medical attention.

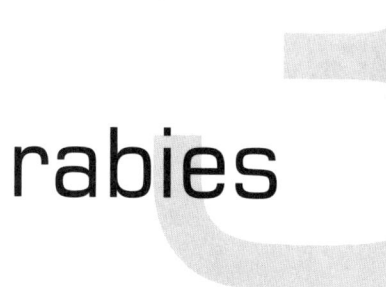

rabies

RABIES – RARE, BUT UNIVERSALLY FATAL

In a Texas hospital, an organ donor died after a brain hemorrhage. Compassionately, his family donated his organs to four different recipients in Texas and Arkansas. Those four people died shortly after the transplants. Why such a tragic loss? Rabies infection.

This was the first known case of someone dying from a transplant of an organ infected with rabies, and measures have been taken since then to ensure the incident is not repeated. Unfortunately, this example illustrates just how dangerous rabies infections can be – to your pets and to you.

Fortunately, there are successful prevention and immunization procedures in place in the United States, and rabies deaths have been limited to one or two annually.

WHAT IS RABIES? Rabies is an acute viral infection that infects the brain and nervous system. When a human experiences a full blown infection, death will occur. An infection of the brain is called an encephalopathy. In addition to the brain infection, muscle spasm or weakness will occur.

HOW DOES THIS OCCUR? Rabies infection is transmitted in the saliva of infected mammals. Most specifically, the carriers of a rabies virus are raccoons, skunks, bats, foxes and coyotes. Domesticated animals such as dogs and cats become infected through close contact and exposure to these other animals. These domestic animals are at risk when they have not received their appropriate shots in order to prevent the development of the disease. It is rare to see rabies in rabbits, squirrels, rats or possums.

For humans, it is dangerous to be in contact with animals that have a high incidence of rabies. Exposure to infected saliva, possibly through a bite, will require immediate medical attention. A human can thus become infected when this infected saliva penetrates broken skin.

VIRAL

WHAT ARE THE SYMPTOMS? Once a human is bitten or exposed, it may take one to three months before symptoms occur. Initially, a person may feel like they have a common cold with stomach flu and fever. There may be a headache with generalized aches and pains. Eventually, a person will have difficulty with muscle control and thought processes. This may lead to hallucinations, agitation and paralysis. Because the person will lose muscle power, they will be unable to breathe and go into cardiac arrest, leading to death.

The initial symptoms are very general and must be correlated with a definite exposure to a rabid animal. This is an important part of the history, so do not be alarmed when you develop generalized flu symptoms without any known exposure to a rabid animal!

HOW IS RABIES DIAGNOSED? Initially, rabies is diagnosed on the basis of history and exposure risks. If exposed to an animal that has a high risk of rabies, treatment will be initiated. In order to diagnose the presence of the virus in a human, the disease process will be in the late fatal stages. Ultimately, brain tissue will be analyzed to check for the virus.

When exposed to a suspect animal, the animal may be quarantined or destroyed. The brain of the animal will be checked for the rabies virus through a special laboratory procedure.

WHAT IS THE TREATMENT? If you are exposed to a high-risk animal and it is not captured, a series of very successful shots will be ordered. First, if exposed, the wound must be cleansed with soap and water immediately. This helps prevent the spread of the virus and potential infection.

Next, your health care provider will analyze the situation and determine if shots are needed. One dose of rabies immune globulin will be given, followed by five shots of a rabies vaccine. These shots are spaced out over 28 days. The full series must be given if the animal is not caught and observed or tested.

Annually, about 18,000 Americans undergo the rabies vaccination series after exposure. There are only about one or two deaths per year in the United States from rabies. The number of deaths from rabies around the world is much higher due to the lack of appropriate animal and human immunizations.

CAN I PREVENT GETTING RABIES? Yes. Be sure that your animals are immunized. Do not play with unfamiliar animals. Do not touch dead animals. Be sure to report sick appearing animals to the Humane Society, who can accurately assess the health of the animal. Finally, if exposed, cleanse the wound immediately and seek medical attention in a timely fashion. You may prevent a fatal illness!

To Your Health with Dr. Wojo

reye's syndrome

It seems that the winter months are filled with sick children and adults. A large majority of the illnesses are secondary to viruses that can cause upper respiratory and gastrointestinal problems. A very rare, but deadly condition may catch your health care provider off guard. It needs to be considered, especially in ill children that are in the post viral phase. This condition is Reye's Syndrome.

WHAT IS REYE'S SYNDROME? Reye's Syndrome is an illness that can affect all bodily organs, but most specifically the liver and brain. After a viral illness, the liver and brain undergo some changes at the cellular level. Those changes are called fatty infiltration. Reye's usually develops during the recovery phase of a viral illness, such as influenza, a common cold or chicken pox.

R.D.K. Reye first described Reye's syndrome in the 1960s in Australia. It was noted that children, in particular, developed altered states of consciousness and severe vomiting in the post-viral phase. It was later discovered that there was an association with the use of aspirin that seemed to cause the syndrome. Once this was identified, the number of cases worldwide decreased. Unfortunately, there is no known cause for the development of the syndrome other than the association of aspirin usage. It is thought that some patients may have an abnormality in metabolism contributing to this problem.

WHAT ARE THE SYMPTOMS? The most common age group of patients affected is between three to twelve years. As noted, the onset of Reye's occurs after the course of a viral illness. Initially, children will develop protracted vomiting, which is a hallmark of the syndrome. Numerous episodes of vomiting are followed by a change in mental status. This may involve increased sleepiness, lethargy, and difficulty with arousal. Laboratory testing may reveal an elevation in liver enzymes that are diagnosed through blood tests.

Initial behavioral changes may be as minor as irritability, but can be as serious as coma. Use of aspirin is a major risk factor for the development of Reye's, but it is not necessary in order to develop the illness.

HOW COMMON IS REYE'S SYNDROME? In the early 1980s, there were over one five hundred cases annually in the United States. Fortunately, that number has decreased to less than one hundred cases per year because of the identification of associated aspirin usage. Internationally, the number of these cases has decreased as well. Usually, most cases are seen between the months of December through March, when the incidence of most viral illnesses are present.

WHAT IS THE TREATMENT? First and foremost, even though Reye's Syndrome is a rare entity, health care providers must be suspicious when seeing very ill children. They must be very suspicious if this is in the post-viral phase of a respiratory illness, protracted vomiting has occurred and there are associated changes in level of consciousness.

Next, supportive treatment is required involving the administration of fluids. A CT scan of the brain and possibly a spinal tap are necessary, in order to rule out evidence of swelling in the brain or other infections such as meningitis. Most of these children will require transfer to a children's intensive care unit at a tertiary care medical center or specialized pediatrics hospital.

If diagnosed early, there is a 75 percent chance of full recovery. If the diagnosis is delayed, there is a high incidence of death. Cases that are diagnosed in a later stage may involve permanent disability due to brain injury.

WHAT SHOULD I DO? It is essential to remember that a large majority of cases of Reye's have been associated with aspirin. DO NOT give aspirin to children! It is safe to use acetaminophen (Tylenol) and ibuprofen to control fever during a viral illness. Even though it is rare, teenagers and adults can develop Reye's as well. It is important to be suspicious of the disease when serious illness develops. More importantly, see your health care provider with those concerns.

To Your Health with Dr. Wojo

severe accute respiritory syndrome (SARS)

When we think of a virus, the flu virus is the first that comes to mind. How do we project ourselves from a virus when we don't event know where it comes from or how to prevent it? The SARS virus is slowly creeping into the United States, quickly festering throughout the world. Will it find its way to Wisconsin? How can we project ourselves? What precautions do we need to take when we travel?

WHAT IS SARS? SARS stands for Severe Acute Respiratory Syndrome that is a constellation of symptoms that center around a respiratory and flu-like illness. The cause of SARS has been in question, but recent reports from the CDC have identified a virus called coronavirus that is reported in Asia, Europe and North America.

WHAT ARE THE SYMPTOMS? The symptoms of SARS are very nonspecific and may mimic other respiratory illnesses. The illness will usually begin with a fever, which is a temperature greater than $100.4°$ F. Chills may follow the fever. Additionally, a patient may experience a headache and generalized aches and pains. Initially, the respiratory symptoms may be mild.

As the disease process progresses, the patient may develop a dry, nonproductive cough. The respiratory illness will progress to a condition of hypoxia, whereby there is a lack of oxygen in the blood. The most severe patients may need to be placed on a ventilator, accounting for 20 percent of all cases.

The incubation period for SARS is thought to be two to seven days. This means that it may take over a week for someone to develop symptoms after they have been exposed to the virus. It may take longer to develop the dry cough and difficulty breathing, as the progression of the disease may be from three to ten days after the development of the initial symptoms.

WHAT ARE THE RISK FACTORS? The primary risk for the development of SARS is travel in an area that has the disease. Thanks to air travel, we have seen an international spread of the cases. At present, the areas with the most reported cases of SARS include mainland China, Hong Kong, Singapore and Hanoi, Vietnam . Toronto, Canada has also been identified as a high-risk area. At the time of this writing, there have been nearly 250 documented cases in the United States. Wisconsin had one suspected documented case.

VIRAL

HOW DOES IT SPREAD? The spread of SARS occurs through direct human-to-human contact. One travels to an endemic area and then the disease is spread to the person's home environment. People living with a SARS patient are at greatest risk. The other potential methods of spread include touching the skin of SARS patients or utensils they have used. Respiratory droplets can be spread through coughing as well. The ability of SARS to spread via broad general environmental contact is not currently known.

WHAT SHOULD I DO? Most importantly, a health care provider must see a patient that is suspect for SARS. A very accurate and detailed travel history must be obtained. Additionally, a comprehensive physical examination will be performed. Baseline laboratory testing will be completed and a chest x-ray will be obtained. This information will only assess the general health of the patient.

At present, there are no tests that can easily identify SARS. The diagnosis is made on clinical grounds and travel history. The CDC is working on tests that will identify antibodies for the disease. These tests would eventually be run in the United States and internationally.

WHAT IS THE TREATMENT? At present, there is no actual treatment for SARS, with the exception of supportive treatment including intravenous rehydration, fever control and respiratory support. None of the current antiviral agents are effective in treating the disease.

More importantly, the prevention of the spread of the disease is essential. If there is risk of exposure, stringent hygiene must be maintained. This includes possible home quarantine for up to 10 days, frequent hand washing, use of respiratory masks preventing spread of droplets, use of disposable rubber gloves and appropriate disinfection of the home.

WHAT ELSE CAN I DO? It is essential for everyone to remain informed about the changing status of the disease. The CDC maintains surveillance of the spread of the disease and is the most up-to-date source. This information can be found at www.cdc.gov.

As with so many medical conditions, it is important to see your health care provider for evaluation and treatment. In the event that you feel that you have risk factors such as travel into an endemic area, followed by symptoms of a respiratory illness, you must seek medical attention!

warts

Often as summer comes to an end and children return to school, it is quite common that little annoyances begin to appear on their hands and feet. These annoyances that look like cauliflower heads are warts. About 25 percent of all children will encounter a wart during their childhood. They are harmless, but ugly, and quite a hassle to get rid of. However, it has been shown that the body can build immunity against warts.

WHAT CAUSES WARTS? Warts are caused by a virus, and most commonly seen on hands and feet. They may initially appear soft and flat, but may change in appearance.

Common warts look like a small head of cauliflower. They are raised and usually well defined. Many times one can see small blood vessels inside the skin lesion. Warts only affect the outermost layer of skin. They do not grow beneath this layer of skin.

In general, warts grow in warm, moist environments. Warts on the foot are common because daily use breaks down the skin. This makes it easier for the virus to get into the skin and grow. Warts are commonly caught in public showers and around swimming pools.

WHAT SHOULD I DO? If you have a wart, it may be self-limited and go away on its own. However, if your wart does not go away, there are numerous ways to treat it and all treatments seem to be equally effective.

The diagnosis of a wart is made by inspection. Over-the-counter treatments of acid-type products may work, but first, the dead skin must be pared off. This process can be very dangerous, especially in diabetics with poor circulation. One needs to be careful not to cause further damage to the affected area.

If warts are numerous, it is reasonable to visit your doctor. Also, many warts can be painful, especially on the foot. These may need to be treated aggressively and removed.

VIRAL

When you see your doctor, several treatments may be recommended. Treatments may include prescription acid-type medicines, cryotherapy (freezing), medicines that cause blistering, or surgically scraping the wart off the skin, which is called curettage.

WHAT IS THE BEST TREATMENT? There is no treatment that stands out as best. In the emergency department, I favor the use of curettage. I have had excellent results over the years with very few reoccurrences.

If treating with curettage, the wart and surrounding area are numbed. There is a bit of pain during the freezing of the wart. Once the area is numb, the entire wart is cut around the edges and scooped out with a dermal curette, that looks like a little ice cream scooper. The patient has to soak the affected area a couple of times daily for a week until the site is completely healed.

CAN I PREVENT WARTS? Just like with many other conditions, prevention is an important part of treatment. Wearing sandals in public showers and around pools may help. Once you find a wart, it is very important not to pick at it and make it bleed. Bleeding may cause the wart to spread to other parts of your body by touch.

In reality, warts are more of a hassle than a major medical problem. They will often go away on their own. Several treatments are effective, but not one stands out as best. Sometimes due to pain, aggressive treatment may be necessary. As always, it is good to seek medical advice prior to initiating home treatment.

west nile

With all of the new health concerns blanketing the nightly news, it's time to be reminded of a virus that had us all talking in the summer of 1999. We watched as the West Nile virus spread from the east coast in 1999, making its way to Wisconsin with a bang in 2002. One element that makes the West Nile virus unique is that it affects both humans and animals, alike. Who is safe? How can we protect our animals? What is it? Where did it come from? Will it ever go away?

WHAT IS WEST NILE VIRUS? The West Nile virus is an infection that is transmitted through infected mosquitoes. The virus is initially harbored in infected birds and carried to humans by mosquitoes. The virus is not transmitted from human to human.

HOW DO I KNOW IF I HAVE BEEN INFECTED? The signs of West Nile virus are quite general. One patient may experience no symptoms, while another experiences a wide variety of flu-like symptoms.

Symptoms include fever, chills, muscle aches, headache or simply feeling un-well. The symptoms may take between a couple of days or a couple of weeks to show. Usually, people will spontaneously recover within a few days.

Unfortunately, some people with underlying medical problems cannot fight the disease as easily as others. Their condition may progress to encephalitis, which is a swelling of the brain. In addition, they may develop meningitis, an inflam-mation of the lining of the brain and spinal cord. These patients feel miserable and appear quite ill. The telltale symptoms of encephalitis and meningitis are a very bad headache and neck pain. Movement of the neck and legs may worsen the headache. These conditions can be fatal.

WHAT SHOULD I DO? In general, for people with no underlying diseases and who are quite healthy, rest and plenty of fluids are recommended. To control a fever, headache or generalized pains, acetaminophen (Tylenol) and ibuprofen (Advil, Motrin) will work. As a rule, it is always wise to avoid the use of aspirin with viruses. Doing so can be fatal.

VIRAL

For those patients that appear very ill and complain of high fever, severe head-ache, stiff neck and generalized weakness, it is important to visit your doctor or go to the hospital.

WHAT CAN I EXPECT? There is no specific treatment for the West Nile virus. If hospitalized, a patient will receive supportive care, that may include IV fluids, pain management and respiratory care. Secondary infections may also need to be treated.

Usually hospitalized patients have underlying medical problems such as a weak immune system or cardiac and respiratory disease. Most fatalities, as a result of the West Nile virus, have occurred in the elderly.

HOW CAN I PROTECT MYSELF? Prevention is the best method of treatment. To avoid contact with mosquitoes in areas that are known to have the West Nile virus, stay indoors during dawn and dusk, when mosquitoes are most active; wear protective clothing; and most importantly, use insect repellent containing DEET. Thirty percent DEET is safe in adults, but children should not be exposed to repellents with DEET higher than 10 percent.

Protect your home environment by spraying for mosquitoes and eliminating as much standing water as possible. This includes puddles, bird baths, plugged rain gutters or containers with water. All of these areas are breeding grounds for mosquitoes.

SHOULD I GET VACCINATED? At present, there is no effective vaccina-tion to prevent the disease. Ongoing research is continuing in this area.

The West Nile virus can have serious consequences for infected patients with chronic underlying medical problems. However, in general, healthy people are not severely affected. Considering the number of mosquito bites that are encountered in the summer months, the rate of West Nile infections is actually very small. Prevention and common sense are important in dealing with this virus. As always, if you have questions, see your doctor.

zoster

I frequently evaluate patients in the emergency department with shingles and the presentation can be varied. In the United States, there are about 500,000 cases of this infectious disease that presents with skin manifestations and pain.

WHAT ARE SHINGLES? This is a skin infection that is caused by the same virus that causes chickenpox. The virus is in the herpes family, called herpes zoster. Herpes comes from the Greek translation of "herpein," which means to creep. This is not associated with a sexually transmitted disease.

Shingles will only occur if someone has had chickenpox. Usually, chickenpox occurs in young patients and shingles in older individuals. The virus may lie dormant for years in a nerve and then it may activate itself. It is not really clear what causes the virus to be activated. Individuals who are immunocompromised with cancer or chronic disease are at greater risk for the development of shingles. Some medicines can put a patient more at risk, as well as the aging process. Stress may also be a factor.

WHAT ARE THE SYMPTOMS? I always remember the case right after I started in the emergency department where a man in his eighties presented and told me that he felt like there were bugs crawling on one side of his forehead. I could not see anything, so I wanted to call the psychiatrist. Luckily I did not, because he came back a few days later with a bunch of blisters on half of his forehead.

One of the first signs of shingles is an abnormal skin sensation. There may be some pain and burning with no physical signs. The location can be anywhere, but we frequently see it on the face, trunk, back and abdomen.

Some patients may be quite sick with fever and chills. There may be some nausea as well and people may just not feel like themselves. Then, the classic rash will appear and diagnosis is made.

The rash may be itchy and it will have blisters. The clear, yellowish, fluid-filled rash will usually be on a reddened skin base. Eventually, the blisters will dry and crust over. The scab will fall off in a few days and there may be a scar left in the area. Many times, the scar and darkened skin will resolve in a few months.

VIRAL

The virus lives in nerves and the line of blisters will be along nerve lines. Thus, the blisters will not cross the midline of the body. So, the rash will usually be on one side of the abdomen, back or face. The rash is very dangerous when it is on the face, as the eye can become involved, resulting in blindness.

People always wonder if shingles are contagious and they are not. But, if you have not had chickenpox, you will get shingles from the blister fluid if you come in contact with it. Direct contact must occur in order to develop the infection.

WHAT SHOULD BE DONE WHEN INFECTED? Shingles is a common medical problem, but medical attention is essential. Many times, the diagnosis is clinical and does not require any testing. The blister fluid can be cultured in the lab in order to make the diagnosis if necessary.

It is best to start treatment within 24 to 48 hours after the blisters appear. Cool compresses may help with the pain. Your health care provider may prescribe an anti-viral medication such as acyclovir that will shorten the course of the illness. This is an oral medication, as the topical medications have less success.

The medical literature has shown that the sooner the treatment, the better the result. A risk is a post-infection pain that is quite severe and called post-herpetic neuralgia. This can lead to a long-term problem with chronic pain at the site.

Shingles is a fairly common problem with a good treatment plan. If you develop shingles, you need to seek medical attention. The severity of the course can be diminished, pain can be reduced and complications can be prevented.

aviation medical examiner (AME)

A highlight of my year is attending the Experimental Aircraft Association Air Adventure in Oshkosh. For aviators and non aviators, we are very fortunate to have the world's largest aviation convention in our backyard. People travel from all over the world to attend the convention that is a trade show, airplane display, air show and aviation educational program. Each year, there are a wide variety of activities that would appeal to just about anyone during the one-week extravaganza.

Over the past few years, I have become a very active pilot holding an instrument rating and commercial pilot license. I fly several times per week as part of my medical legal consulting practice and share two V-Tail Bonanza single engine airplanes. Most recently, I spent a week in Oklahoma City with the Federal Aviation Association becoming certified as an Aviation Medical Examiner (AME). I am the only one in my county authorized by the FAA to perform aviation medical examinations.

You may not be aware of this, but all pilots must hold a valid aviation medical card in order to pilot an airplane. Let's look into the process of the aviation medical exam and see what sort of medical conditions may disqualify a pilot from flying.

WHAT IS AN AME? In the United States, an AME is a physician that is authorized by the FAA to perform physical examinations and issue airman medical certificates. These physicians are not employees of the FAA, but selected by the regional office and thus trained. It is not a requirement for the physician to be a pilot, but it is preferred.

Initially, an AME can issue a Second or Third Class certificate. A First Class certificate can only be issued by a Senior AME who has completed flight physicals for at least three years and received the additional FAA designation.

WHAT ARE PILOT PHYSICALS? The FAA has designed three classes of pilot physicals. A First Class medical certificate is required for individuals that act as pilot-in-command of an air carrier flight or some charter flights. This examination includes an EKG and must be repeated every six months.

WELLNESS

The Second Class medical certificate is required of any commercial pilot that is operating an aircraft for compensation. This would include cargo pilots, crop dusters and banner towers. In addition, a corporate pilot may fall under this category. This examination is valid for one year.

The Third Class medical certificate is the most common of all certificates for private pilots. It is valid for two years for individuals over 40 years and three years if the age is less than 40.

The physical examination for all classes is the same, as well as many of the guidelines. A comprehensive head-to-toe exam is completed. Vision must be 20/20 corrected. Hearing must be adequate. Color blindness is assessed. Blood pressure must be less than 155/95. There must be no history of psychiatric illness or substance abuse.

If a pilot does not meet the requirements, the results of the examination are deferred to a panel of specialist physicians in Oklahoma City at the FAA. A special issuance may be given for certain conditions. Many times, restrictions on aircraft operation may be in place.

Certain medications may disqualify a pilot as well. The FAA has a large list of medications that cannot be taken while operating an aircraft. Most of this information can be found at www.faa.org. This is a useful website that has information about pilots, airplanes and training.

Even though the process is quite stringent, the FAA and the AME want every pilot to pass their physical. It is important to note that this process is to ensure the safety of the pilot, passengers and the general public.

My week in Oklahoma City exposed me to a great deal of information and I was very impressed with the amount of research that occurs at the FAA. It was reassuring to see that all of the rules and regulations are developed on the basis of very extensive research data, and not just on arbitrary information. Aviation is a wonderful profession and hobby, so I would encourage those who are interested to learn to fly.

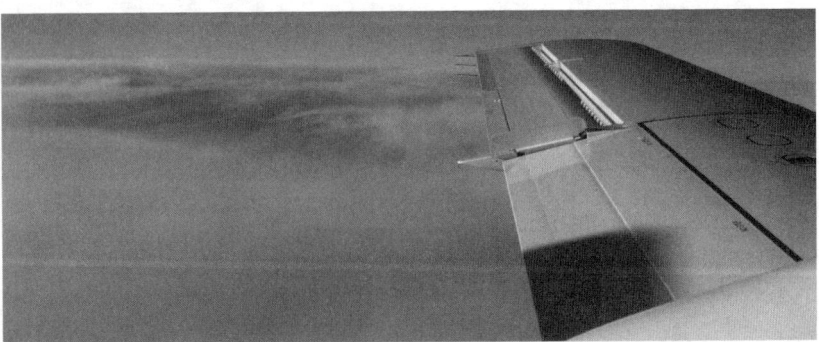

botox

Mirror, mirror on the wall, how can I have the youngest looking face of them all? In the past women wanting a wrinkle-free face would reach for little strips of tape that would be placed on the temple and into the hairline. The result was their crows feet disappeared and they had a smoother-looking face, but when used, women needed to be careful how they turned their face so that their friends would not see their little hidden secret. Now, fast forward to 2003 where women and men alike are receiving injections of Botox for that flawless-looking face. When done correctly you can lose almost 20 years off of your appearance, but when overdone, two words come to mind…Joan Rivers.

WHAT IS BOTOX? Botox is a manufactured toxin that comes from botulism, a form of food poisoning that causes paralysis and death. There are several different strains of Clostridium botulinum that release toxins classified as A through G. Botox is a Type A toxin that has been used medically for years.

This Type A toxin has been primarily used when treating painful muscle spasms, most commonly in the neck. The muscle, when injected, would become paralyzed for about three months, relieving this painful debilitating condition. In addition, Botox was often used for treating children with a lazy eye.

Most recently, it was found that small doses carefully injected into a specific muscle around wrinkle lines, would paralyze the underlying muscle and smooth out the skin. The results were obvious shortly after the injection.

WHAT IS THE PROCEDURE? Physicians, primarily plastic surgeons, have been trained in the use of Botox. They have been able to identify areas on the face where the injection will help improve appearance. Once the areas of facial rejuvenation have been identified and marked, the simple injection process begins.

Botox is injected into the defined area using a very small 30-gauge needle. The patient may begin to experience some discomfort at the site of the injection, but this is brief. Ice is then applied to those injected areas in order to decrease the incidence of swelling and bruising. It may take a few days to see the results, but the underlying small facial muscles will be chemically paralyzed for a period of up to five months.

WHAT ARE THE COMPLICATIONS? In general, complications are somewhat rare and usually minor. As noted in medical literature there are no reported allergic reactions as a direct result of receiving Botox injections. In some cases, a patient may experience some localized redness or bruising. Before receiving Botox injections it is very important to inform your doctor regarding the use of aspirin or Coumadin, drugs that thin the blood and can cause bleeding.

Additionally, paralysis of surrounding muscles can occur. It has been noted that when "crows feet" around the eyes are injected, a patient may develop a drooping of the eyelid. This side effect is rather short lived.

IS BOTOX SAFE? Botox has been used medically in qualified hands since 1980 with minimal side effects. Two Canadian physicians in the mid-1990s pioneered the use in cosmetic surgery and numerous medical articles have been published in support of its use.

One complication that has been cited in a few instances is headaches. In the January 2002 issue of the Journal of the American Academy of Dermatology, an article was published focusing on Botox entitled "Severe, Intractable Headaches After Injections with Botulism A Exotoxin." The story mentioned four cases of the complication, which would make up roughly one percent of all the patients studied.

WHAT SHOULD I DO? In the event that you decide to undergo this procedure, you must seek out a very qualified and experienced physician. This practitioner must have a proven track record and a detailed understanding of facial musculature and architecture. The procedure should be completed in an accomplished medical facility. Seek out recommendations from other patients who have undergone the procedure. Be sure to investigate the cost, as most insurance companies will not cover this expense and even though it is cheaper than surgery, the injections are quite costly.

Headphones and hearing loss

As a Mac user since the 1980s, it has been pretty cool to watch the progression of technology, especially with Apple. Since I have to personally work in a fairly quiet environment, especially when writing, I do not own an iPod, but these devices have stormed the nation as music players and media storage devices.

I read with interest a study that was released from Northwestern University's Department of Communication Sciences and Disorders Department. The study revealed that our youth are ruining their hearing by listening to their iPods too loudly.

It was also noted that the little ear buds that snuggly fit into the ear canal are the major culprits. These earpieces are placed close to the eardrum with magnified and prolonged sound and can cause hearing loss. This is one of the first studies to specifically look at this, but it has been known since the 1980s that loud music can contribute to hearing loss, especially in concertgoers.

It was shown that the little ear buds increase sound intensity by nine decibels. This is the difference of the sound coming from an alarm clock versus a lawn mower. Since the ear buds do not fit snuggly, the volume must be increased in order to block background noise. Therein lies part of the problem.

Research has shown that the over-the-ear type earphones are safer, but not as convenient. This is something to be considered when outfitting your child or teen with a music player. Also, noise canceling headphones are much better and safer, but more costly.

WHAT ARE THE TYPES OF HEARING LOSS? There are three classifications of hearing loss. Sensorineural loss occurs when there is damage to some of the internal ear structures. Conductive hearing loss is when sound is blocked from coming into the ear, like with earwax. Mixed loss is a combination of the above.

WHAT CAUSES HEARING LOSS? There are several causes including birth defects, infection, trauma and tumors. Some side effects of medication may lead to hearing loss as well. Each cause needs to be investigated.

WELLNESS

HOW IS THIS DIAGNOSED? In the event that hearing loss is experienced, a medical professional must investigate it. A physician specializing in otorhinolaryngology or Ears-Nose-Throat (ENT) should evaluate the problem. Hearing tests and an evaluation by an audiologist or hearing specialist will be in order. The type and severity of the hearing loss will be determined and recommendations for treatment will be made depending on the problem.

WHAT ELSE CAN BE DONE? It is essential that our youth understand the dangers of the loud music and hearing loss. They must protect their hearing. The current recommendations for the iPod include a 60/60 rule or a 60/30 rule.

The 60/60 rule applies if music is being listened to with an over-the-ear headset. The volume of the MP3 player should be at a maximum of 60 percent and listened to for a total of 60 minutes per day.

If ear buds are used, the 60/30 rule applies. The volume should be no greater than 60 percent of maximum and the music should be listened to for up to 30 minutes per day. These recommendations should be followed, as this is the best way to prevent lifelong hearing loss that cannot be reversed. Encourage our youth to follow these guidelines and set an example if you own an iPod or other personal MP3 player.

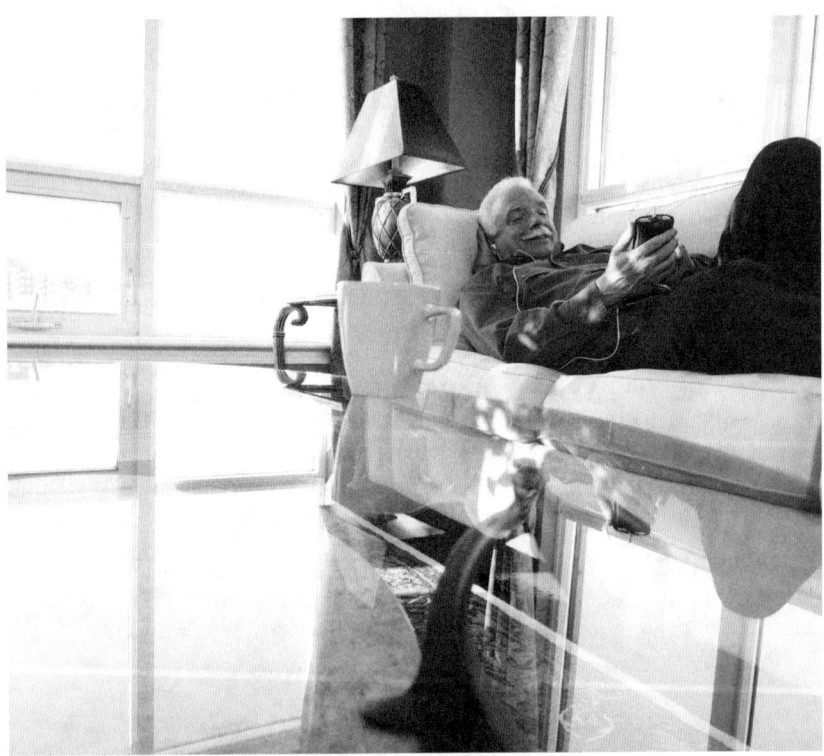

lasik

Are you tired of wearing glasses? Can't see well through the fog on your spectacles when you come in from the cold? Unable to see what time it is when you wake up in the middle of the night? Have some extra cash in your Medical Savings Account? You may want to consider surgical vision correction. Over the past few years, thousands of patients have been successfully treated and are now free of glasses. Let's look a little more closely at surgical visual corrective procedures. The most common procedure is called LASIK.

WHAT IS LASIK? LASIK is a laser vision procedure that is used to primarily correct myopia (near-sightedness), presbyopia (far-sightedness), or astigmatism (unequal vision). LASIK stands for laser in-situ keratomileusis.

This procedure has also been called "flap and zap," because the cornea, which is the clear portion of the eye, is cut and then repositioned. The excess tissue is then very accurately removed, reshaping the eye and correcting the vision. This reshaping actually allows light traveling through the cornea to be properly focused on the retina. The retina is at the back of the eye and it receives the visual image that is interpreted by the brain.

IS THIS THE ONLY PROCEDURE? No. LASIK has been the most common surgical visual correction in recent years. Other procedures that have been used in visual correction include PRK (photorefractive keratectomy) and CR (conductive keratoplasty).

PRK is similar to LASIK, but a flap is not raised on the cornea. The cornea is re-shaped by the laser. With CR, radiowaves are sent along the surface of the cornea, thereby shrinking it. This leads to reshaping of the cornea and correcting the vision. Wavefront technology is now being employed to more accurately restructure the eye, which is done with the LASIK and involves the use of computer imaging. All of the procedures have their merits

WHAT SHOULD I DO? You need to decide if you want to undergo surgical correction of your vision. Most insurance plans do not cover these procedures, so you will incur an out-of-pocket expense that may range from $1500 to $3000 per eye. There are several factors that determine the cost, so this must be discussed with your pre-surgical counselor.

WELLNESS

You will be asked to not wear hard contacts for a couple of weeks prior to surgery. If you wear soft contacts, you will have to wear your glasses for a few days prior to the correction. Your vision needs to be stable for a year prior to surgery and you must be at least 18. Pregnant women must wait until after delivery.

WHAT KIND OF PHYSICIAN DOES THIS SURGERY? It is important to find an ophthalmologist that specializes in these surgical procedures. An ophthalmologist is a physician that specializes in medical and surgical care of the eye.

LASIK is the most common procedure being completed today with very good results. Studies have been shown that about 90 percent of all patients achieve 20/40 vision. Good results have been achieved in carefully selected patients.

DOES THIS REQUIRE HOSPITALIZATION? No. In general, LASIK is an outpatient procedure that is completed within 20 minutes. Local anesthesia is placed in the eye to numb it. Many of these procedures are now completed in the office of the ophthalmologist.

WHAT ARE THE COMPLICATIONS? In general, the complications are minimal and usually short-lived. After the surgery, vision may be clouded while the cornea heals. There may be some problems with night vision and a patient may see halos around light sources. There may also be a temporary intolerance of bright lights.

All of these side effects usually resolve with time. A patient may experience an overcorrection and may need a second surgery, but this is rare. It is important that the patient is healthy and that the eye is free of disease.

WHAT SHOULD I DO? If you feel that you are a suitable candidate for LASIK surgery, you need to meet with your ophthalmologist and discuss the surgical procedures available. LASIK does work and has good results. In addition, the recovery time period is quite short.

low carb diet

If I had a dollar for every time someone came to me with a question about how to lose weight, I would own my own publishing empire. There have been many diet crazes in the past, but we have not seen anything as hot as the Atkins diet. It's so large that food industries such as citrus, bread and potato are changing their advertising campaigns to adjust to the hits their industries have taken. The interesting thing is that one of the last diet fads was the pasta diet, which represented everything the Atkins diet is against.

There is money to be made with these diet crazes as well. Are you aware that the Atkins name now has its own food line? So when you hear diets being "pushed," be careful and listen not just to what those diets can do to your body, good and bad, but look to see who is doing the pushing and who will be making money from these dietary changes.

The Atkins diet was hot in California long before it made its way to Wisconsin. That being said, Californians, and the doctors in California, are now noticing the ramifications that a long-term, high-protein diet can have on your body– particularly your heart. Let's take a closer look at the Atkins diet.

WHAT IS THE ATKINS DIET? Back in the late 1970s, Dr. Robert Atkins, a New York City cardiologist developed a diet plan that focused on the intake of high protein foods, with a restriction of carbohydrates. Foods that are high in protein are all of the meats such as beef, pork, chicken and fish. The only dairy products allowed were eggs and cheese. Complex carbohydrates such as high fiber vegetables were allowed. Breads, pastas and desserts were taboo.

THE RESULT? Dr. Atkins' patients began to lose weight very quickly. Unfortunately for Dr. Atkins, in the late 1970s through the early 1990s, he was considered a heretic. The medical community and the general public had embraced the American Heart Association and the American College of Cardiology's position that the best diet was a low-fat diet that was high in carbohydrates.

The supermarkets were filled with low-fat foods in green boxes. Unfortunately, these foods were very high in carbohydrates. Even though the foods were fairly low in calories, Americans thought that they could over-indulge in these "safe foods." The result? Americans are now 20 percent heavier on average than 25 years ago.

WELLNESS

WAS DR. ATKINS WRONG? No. Recent medical research has shown that there was merit to the thought process developed by Dr. Atkins. A small study has shown that when a group of dieters on the high-protein, low-carbohydrate diet were compared to low-fat intake dieters, the high-protein folks lost about nine more pounds than the other study group. The medical community has embraced the high protein diet for a short period of weight loss for up to six months.

ATKINS VERSUS SOUTH BEACH DIET? In 2003, Dr. Arthur Agatston, a Miami cardiologist, published his successful diet program that he had been recommending for years. This diet has been an instant success and his book has spent weeks on the New York Times Best Seller list. Some people refer to his program as "Atkins Lite."

The South Beach diet focuses on a high protein diet that is low in carbohydrates. Dr. Agatston recommends high protein foods that are lower in fat content. He is not as strict about reducing carbohydrates, but defines good and bad carbohydrates. He recommends a variety of vegetables initially, and after the first two weeks, more carbohydrates can be added. Overall, he views this as a change in lifestyle. The principle behind both diets is that the high protein foods provide longer satiation and therefore, there is less caloric intake. The scientific principles behind both diets do have merit.

WHAT ABOUT LOW CARBOHYDRATE FOODS? Just like the 20-year craze for low fat foods in green boxes, low carbohydrate foods are starting to flood the market. Many of these foods are good, but they are not a free ticket to over-indulge. It is good that the carbohydrate content has been analyzed, but there are still some issues.

Recently, many foods are marketed as "low net-carbs." The food companies have changed their processing of many of the foods and added sugar alcohols and fibers. The content of these two elements are subtracted from the total content of carbohydrate in the food. This may be a marketing gimmick, so be careful! This concept is being currently studied and analyzed. The government may need to intervene on this labeling issue if the actual content is not accurately represented.

WHAT SHOULD I DO? Weight loss is important in maintaining a healthy lifestyle and reducing disease such as heart attacks and strokes. Moderation and exercise are two very important elements to a successful weight-loss program. Both of these diets have scientific merit, but it is important to consult a health care provider to assist in choosing a safe weight loss program that will have long-term results.

seatbelts

Automobile accidents are a reality. The best way to keep yourself safe is to buckle up. If you don't, you risk being catapulted from your car or crushed– among other things. Let's look a little more closely at the issues surrounding seatbelt usage.

WHY ARE SEATBELTS IMPORTANT? The most common cause of accidental death in the United States is trauma suffered during a motor vehicle accident. About 50,000 Americans die each year from injuries sustained in a motor vehicle accident, and over 4 million victims sustain an injury in an auto crash.

In Wisconsin, it is the law that seatbelts must be worn. In 2000, nearly 12,000 lives were saved as the direct result of seat belt usage. The chances of surviving a severe auto accident are improved by nearly 50 percent by simply wearing a seatbelt. The chances of surviving a light truck crash are improved by over 60 percent when you are belted in that vehicle.

WHAT ARE COMMON INJURIES? The type of motor vehicle accident will determine the type of injury a victim will sustain. Head-on collisions cause significant head, neck, chest, abdominal and extremity injuries. Broad side accidents contribute to a great deal of internal organ damage and pelvis/hip injuries. Rear end crashes may injure a patient's neck, back and chest. It is important for the health care provider to be apprised of the mechanism of injury. This will aid in an appropriate and expedient diagnosis.

Unrestrained vehicle occupants are frequently ejected from the vehicle and 75 percent of all motor vehicle fatalities involve a victim being ejected. Only 1 percent of all people report being belted and then ejected from their auto or truck. A victim that has been ejected frequently suffers severe head and body trauma. In addition, this victim is at risk for severe internal injuries such as a ruptured spleen, lacerated liver or a ruptured aorta. Most of the victims never make it to the emergency department alive.

WHY SHOULD SEATBELTS BE WORN AT ALL TIMES? About 75 percent of all auto accidents happen within a 25-mile radius of one's home. About 80 percent of all accidents happen at a speed of 40 mph or less. Victims in crashes of 10 mph have been killed. You have a 25-fold increase in being killed if thrown out of your vehicle. Did you know that most Americans will be involved in one crash every 10 years? It is essential to remember that the driver and passenger cannot control the actions of other vehicles and drivers.

WHAT SHOULD I DO? Everyone, young and old must wear a seatbelt at all times when in a motor vehicle. Wisconsin is one of 49 states that require all occupants to be belted in a moving vehicle. New Hampshire is the only state that has not adopted this legislation.

Primary seatbelt laws allow one to be cited for not wearing a seatbelt if observed by law enforcement. Secondary seatbelt laws only allow for legal citations if another motor vehicle infraction is noted at the time of the stop. Research has shown that the primary seatbelt laws have increased the usage of seatbelts and lives have been saved.

It is really important that seatbelts be worn at all times. Contrary to the argument that one will be trapped in a burning or submerged auto, the death rate is still significantly lower for victims involved in these accidents if seatbelts are worn. Also, these types of accidents are quite rare.

Overall, the safety and medical literature have clearly shown over the years that the increased usage of seatbelts has improved the chances of surviving a severe auto crash. It has also been shown that the chance for permanent disability is significantly decreased with the consistent wearing of shoulder and lap belts. Why take a chance?

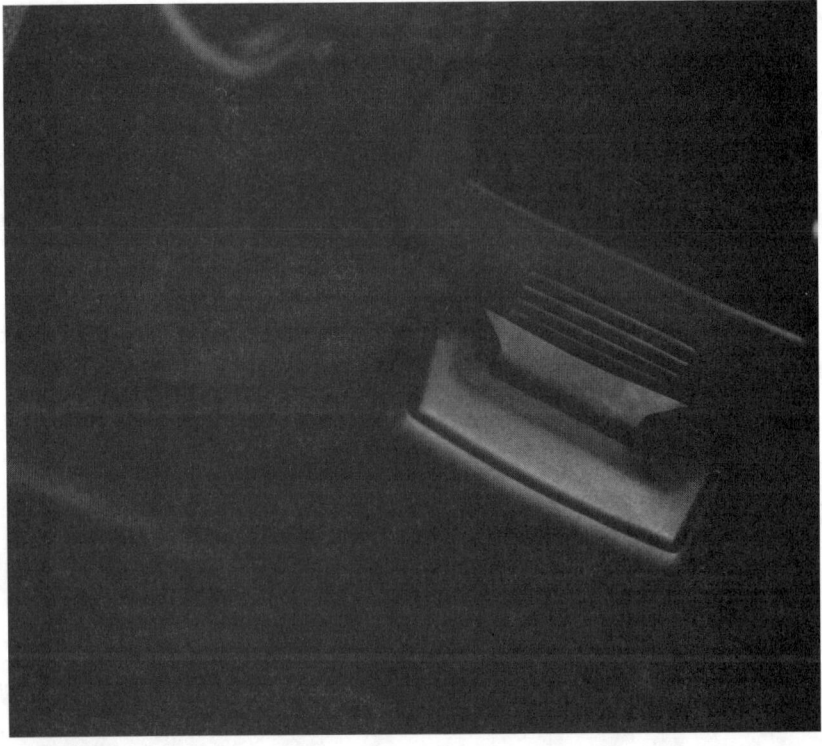

sunburn

Do you remember in the 70s, when your sister would put on the cocoa butter and lay out in the sun for hours? She and her friends would have contests to see who could get a better (which meant deeper in color) tan. Fast forward ten years to when tanning beds came along, and it seemed that the only drawback were the two pressure points that never seemed to tan on your shoulder blades. That was then. Now we have sun block with 50 SPF and countries such as Australia implementing "no hat no play" regulations for children. Tans look great, but as we all know, can be deadly. Like many other cosmetic benefits, what is the price we pay for looking good? Death?

WHAT IS SUNBURN? Sunburn is actually a first-degree burn of the skin that is caused by over-exposure to the sun. The ultraviolet rays of the sun, which penetrate even clouds, cause the burn. More than 75 percent of our nation's children have experienced at least one sunburn, and more than 50 percent have had at least three or more sunburns in one summer.

WHAT ARE THE SYMPTOMS? The common symptoms of sunburn include generalized redness, pain, possible blistering in severe cases, itching and generalized warmth to the skin. Some severe cases may also present significant swelling of the skin, most notable on the face.

HOW IS IT TREATED? As with any burn, the first step is to remove the patient from the offending environment. So, get out of the sun into a cool environment. Next, begin cooling the skin with water. It is important to not cause an episode of hypothermia (lowering of the core body temperature). This treatment may last several minutes to an hour.

Oral pain medication should be used. Studies have shown that the use of aspirin has decreased pain and inflammation to a significant degree. Other over-the-counter medications such as acetaminophen (Tylenol) and ibuprofen (Motrin, Advil) usually work well too.

It is important not to use grease salves and ointments on a new burn. This may inhibit the healing process and trap the heat of the skin over the burn. Eventually, over-the-counter one percent hydrocortisone cream may be applied in a very thin layer to the burned skin.

HOW LONG WILL THIS LAST? In general, the severe symptoms of sunburn will last from 24 to 48 hours. This will eventually lead to skin peeling and itching. At this time, it is important to keep the skin well hydrated with skin moisturizers and lotions. It is really important not to re-expose the skin to the effects of the sun during the healing period.

WHAT ELSE SHOULD I DO? Prevention is the key. Sunburn is associated with significant delayed health risks. The development of malignant melanoma is directly related to sun-damaged skin. Malignant melanoma is a very aggressive skin cancer that has a very high mortality rate.

It is very important to protect children from the sunlight. Medical studies have shown that sunburned parents usually have sunburned children. There is a direct correlation to the amount of sunscreen use between parents and children.

It is essential to limit exposure of the sun by children during the times of 10 a.m. and 4 p.m. All children should have a 15 SPF or higher sunscreen applied. The use of protective clothing is essential as well.

IS THERE ANYTHING ELSE? It is really important that parents educate their children on the dangers of over-exposure to the sun. It may be hard for children to understand that their actions may have significant long-term health consequences as they age. Be sure to provide a safe environment for your children to play in and encourage healthy living at an earlier age!

supplements

One pill, two pill, three pill, four...there is a pill for everything. Want to think more clearly? Pop a pill. Sleep longer? Take two. Wake up quicker? Take one and wash it down with a cup of coffee. Then, there is the weight-loss struggle. The standard for that is a program of two pills, three times a day, before every meal.

But are these "remedies" being regulated appropriately or at all, for that matter? Hopefully we have all learned what the misuse of Ephedra can do, but how many other drugs are out there that are quietly killing people?

It seems that there has been little control of the herbal and natural supplement industry. Congress is now calling for the implementation of much stricter guidelines that regulate the research, distribution and sale of herbal, natural and dietary supplements.

WHAT IS A SUPPLEMENT? Supplements and vitamins are substances that occur naturally in the body and the environment. Vitamins present in the body include A, B, C, D, E and K. In addition, there are herbal medicines that are naturally grown substances that are thought to have some medicinal and therapeutic value. These substances are not considered part of Western mainstream medicine and are referred to as alternative or contemporary medicine.

IS THIS A COMMON PRACTICE? Over the years, the use and acceptance of vitamins and supplements has grown significantly. It has been estimated that about one-third of all Americans have used some form of supplementation in their lifetime. More than three billion dollars are spent annually on supplements and this is increasing about 10 percent annually.

Many patients that use supplements are not dissatisfied with Western medicine, but they are looking for an enhancement to their life. Physicians and other health care providers have begun to embrace the use of supplementation and many medical schools are offering courses on herbal medicine. It is important for providers to understand what their patients are taking and the merits of the herbal medicine or vitamin.

WELLNESS

ARE SUPPLEMENTS AND VITAMINS SAFE? There are several issues that surround these questions. Just because something is naturally occurring does not mean it is safe. The body maintains a balance of vitamins with an appropriate well-balanced diet. Some medical conditions such as pregnancy, dietary problems or alcoholism require vitamin supplementation.

As with Ephedra, there are several herbal medications that may be dangerous to the body directly or through an interaction with another prescribed medication. Recently, Aristolochia has been shown to cause kidney problems. Some of the naturally occurring hormones such as Androstenedione (Andro) that are used by athletes have been linked to cancer and liver disease.

With the absence of Ephedra, many dietary and weight-loss products have begun to use Bitter Orange, which is another type of stimulant. This stimulant, just like Ephedra, has been linked to heart disease, high blood pressure and stroke. A problem that has been identified with many of these substances involves the quality control of the manufacturing process. The FDA monitors this process as it does with other prescribed pharmaceuticals.

WHAT SHOULD I DO? As health care providers, we are cautious in recommending supplements until research has adequately investigated the actions of the medications and their side effects. It is essential to do your own research on these products, if you choose to take them. Internet and literature searches must be limited to peer reviewed sites that are evidence-based. This means that there has been research that supports or discourages their use. The medical sites should be affiliated with an academic center or government agency.

Be sure to stay away from some of the supplements that are now in question. Let your health care provider know if you are taking any of these products, as several drug interactions can occur with your prescribed pharmaceuticals. Limit your intake of supplements and vitamins, as this can be very costly and dangerous.

At this time, stay away from "weight loss" supplements, as there is controversy over the safety and efficacy of these products. Many of the side effects can be deadly. Be sure to report any side effect to your doctor and the FDA. This is very important information that may help others as well.

violence

When people hear that I have practiced emergency medicine for nearly 20 years, they comment that I must have some amazing experiences and stories. Well, I certainly have seen a lot of different things over the past years. The practice of emergency medicine has changed since I started and it continues to change.

Most importantly, the quality of care that is administered in our emergency department, as well as most community hospitals, has improved. We are involved in a variety of national quality initiatives and monitor our practices on a daily basis. We not only look at what treatment modalities are the best, but at how we can deliver the therapeutics in the most efficient and cost-effective way. Thus, as a patient, you benefit from the most current plans of care that are based on the research in medicine.

The practice has also changed in our community and across the country. A large percentage of our patients are elderly with complex medical problems. As we continue to live longer, medical problems and complications arise with an increase in age. Thus, a majority of our day is spent trying to figure out some of the consequences of the aging process.

With the advent of trauma systems, many community emergency departments, such as the one I work in, have seen less major trauma patients. Research has shown that patients benefit most at a designated trauma center with a variety of resources. As with anything, more resources lead to a better outcome. It has been shown that a major trauma patient that is managed in a hospital with a designated trauma program will have a more successful recovery. This is due to the availability of multiple medical specialties and support systems.

In addition, the types of trauma cases have diminished over the years. Better and safer automobiles have lead to less injury. There is no question that the tougher drunk driving laws and awareness lead to less injury as well. Years ago, I could always anticipate on having to deal with a major motor vehicle crash related to alcohol every weekend that I worked. Fortunately, that does not seem to be the case any longer. Drivers are more conscientious about this issue, but the problem has not gone away.

Unfortunately, a large percentage of trauma cases that we still see are secondary to violence and this has not changed much over the past several years. Large portions of the violent acts that result in trauma are alcohol and drug-related. Surprisingly, almost any day of the week, we see people that are impaired and involved in a violent act.

Violence can be directed at one's self, and other people such as children, spouses and the elderly. Many of these acts lead to serious physical injuries and mental scarring. When these acts involve a child or an elder, the law requires that we report this to legal authorities and social services. As a health care professional, it is not my place to make a judgment, but we must have the situation investigated to protect those involved. Violence may also be directed at personal property. All of these problems tax our resources. Many of these cases end up in the emergency department for treatment.

Impairment from drugs and alcohol may lead to senseless acts. We spend a great deal of time patching up folks involved in physical altercations or loss of coordination while trying to perform physical tasks. It is hard to believe that people decide to fix their roof after they are under the influence! Alcohol is not the only culprit that leads to violent acts. Methamphetamine or "meth", crack cocaine, and marijuana are other big players in large and small communities.

Fortunately, in central Wisconsin, our problems are small compared to the major metropolitan areas. We have a strong medical, legal, educational and social community that is fairly well-equipped to deal with these problems. Most importantly, awareness of the problem and the ability to address it is essential in improving the quality of life for all of our residents, especially our children and youth.

walking

Over the past 20 years, my parents have been involved in a daily walking program. Most people in their rural neighborhood know them and see them out pounding the pavement almost every day of the year. Granted, the weather in central Wisconsin is not always conducive to their activity, but they usually find a way to get in their daily trek, which is usually over three miles. They are both in their mid-seventies, and this has certainly kept them physically and mentally fit.

Walking is a great way to exercise and stay healthy. Numerous medical studies have shown that walking leads to a lower incidence of heart disease, cancer and other chronic illnesses. This is an athletic activity that requires minimal equipment– just a good pair of shoes! It is an excellent physical activity for all ages.

WHAT ARE THE BENEFITS? Research has shown that prevention of numerous medical problems can occur through a dedicated walking program. For example, increasing physical activity leads to weight reduction. This leads to improved cardiovascular health and prevention of heart attacks. Through weight reduction and exercise, there is a decreased risk for the development of adult onset diabetes. In addition, lung capacity is improved and you will feel better.

With the aging process, osteoporosis (thinning of the bones) is always a worry. Exercise has been shown to keep bones strong and healthy. This leads to a decreased risk of fractures, such as a broken hip. When the hip breaks with thinned bones, it usually occurs before the fall. Also, if a fall does occur and the bones are strong, there is less chance of a fracture.

WHAT INJURIES OCCUR? The risks of injuries are usually secondary to overuse or direct trauma. As with most conditions, prevention is the best medicine.

Be sure to keep yourself safe from direct trauma. Wear appropriate clothing that is bright and easily seen by motorists during the day or night. Being struck by a car can cause significant injury, disability or death. Know your route and carry a cell phone if possible.

Previously, I wrote about overuse injuries in student athletes and focused on plantar fasciitis and shin splints. This can turn into a chronic problem and both conditions get better with rest. Plantar fasciitis presents as a painful arch and heel, while shin splints present with pain over the shinbone. Good shoe gear and avoidance of excessive walking can prevent the development of this problem.

It is important to wear good, stable shoes that are well padded. Many times, your local shoe store has trained and certified employees in pedorthics. These individuals are able to help analyze your foot structure and gait, and determine which shoe is best. The fit not only affects motion of the foot and ankle, but also leads to improved comfort.

Poorly fitted shoes can lead to blisters and "black toe." If you develop a blister and it is large, it may help to have it drained at the base of the blister. This will prevent it popping and peeling off. The layer of skin will protect the under layer and it will be less painful. Eventually, the top layer will dry up and fall off.

With a tight shoe, the big toenail can become bruised and there may even be a collection of blood under the nail. This can be painful and the nail may fall off. This is also a common problem in marathon runners or people who participate in long walks that are the length of a marathon.

WHAT ELSE SHOULD I DO? Most walking injuries are minor in nature and usually due to poor conditioning and overuse. The standard orthopedic treatment measures are best including rest, ice, compression and elevation, known as RICE therapy. Use of ibuprofen and Tylenol will help with the aches and pains, as well as inflammation.

Most importantly, start gradually and work your way up. Be sure to have medical clearance from your health care provider prior to starting. Also, if you have questions about getting started, your health care provider, athletic trainer or physical therapist is a great resource. It is always important to seek medical advice if a problem arises. Walking is a tremendous way to stay healthy and live longer!

water safety

WATER SAFETY STARTS AT HOME – KNOW YOUR LIMITS AND CPR

Did you know that the summer months are the most dangerous months for children? Safety, especially water safety, becomes ever more important this time of year.

Nationally, more than 3 million emergency department visits involve children who have suffered a traumatic event like drowning. Sadly, studies confirm that 90 percent of all of these accidents are preventable.

Unintentional injury is the number one killer of children– exceeding disease, violence and suicide. Hopefully, with proper safety knowledge and an awareness of our surroundings, we can prevent an accidental water death this summer.

HOW COMMON IS DROWNING? Drowning is the second leading cause of unintentional death in children, only secondary to motor vehicle trauma. Nearly 1,000 children drown each year in the United States and about 4,000 children are hospitalized after a near drowning event. Unfortunately, a majority of these cases could have been prevented.

A recent SAFE KIDS study did show that 90 percent of children that drowned were being supervised. It has been shown that parents that supervise their children do simultaneously participate in other activities such as talking to someone, reading, eating and using the phone. It only takes a minute for tragedy to strike and it is imperative to closely supervise children.

WHAT SHOULD PARENTS DO? There are four water safety wisdoms recommended. Supervision by a designated adult is essential and there should be no distractions. Adults may wish to work in shifts in order to actively supervise water activities. Secondly, the environment around pools must be safe. Safety in these areas includes the use of pool covers, appropriate fencing and alarms. Home pools must be child proofed so that a child may not accidentally get into a pool area unsupervised.

A third recommendation is the use of appropriate safety gear. Children must wear U.S. Coast Guard life vests when in and around the water. In addition, many states require children to wear a life vest when in a boat at all times. The use of life vests has shown to prevent 85 percent of all boat-related drownings. Lastly, educating children about the dangers of the water is critical. All children should have gone through swimming lessons by the age of eight. It has been shown that nearly three-fourths of all children that drown did not know how to swim.

WHAT ELSE CAN BE DONE? The SAFE KIDS campaign has other common sense recommendations for adults and children. It is important that adults never let children swim alone. Unsafe activities should be discouraged such as running and pushing.

Adults should educate themselves with emergency procedures such as infant and child CPR. This training prepares the adult to deal with an emergency situation appropriately. More importantly, it is essential to prevent two drownings by throwing a flotation device or using a reaching device in order to rescue a child, as opposed to jumping in. This also prevents neck injuries in those who dive in prior to adequately assessing the surroundings. Lastly, "water wings" and inflatable inner tubes are not safety devices.

WHAT SHOULD CHILDREN DO? Children must be informed about the dangers of the water and they must learn to swim. They must always swim with a buddy. They must be taught to not push others in the water and act responsibly. Parents should set the standard that a life vest must be worn at all times when around the water and this policy must be adhered to 100 percent of the time. Lastly, it is important that children swim in appropriate designated areas of lakes, rivers and oceans.

Summer is a wonderful time of the year for family activities. Please take the time to encourage and provide a safe environment for your children.

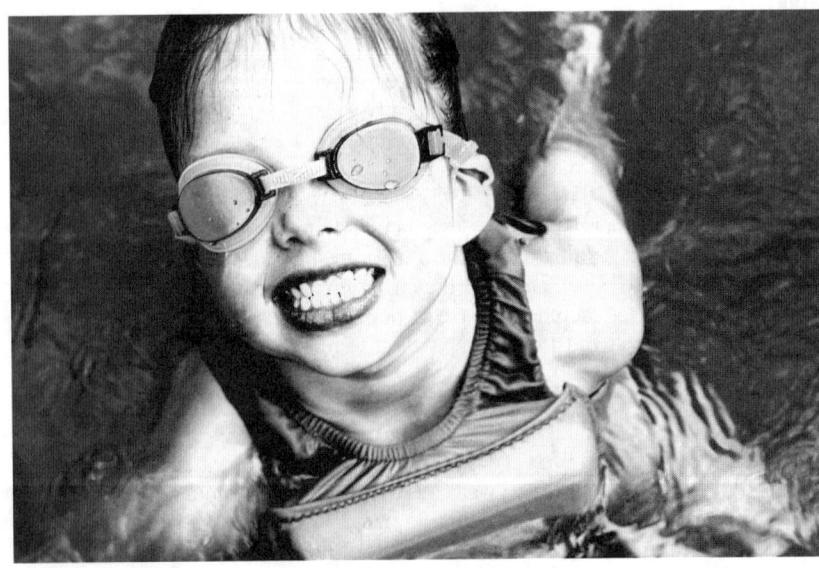

weight loss surgery

Atkins, South Beach, The Zone, and Weight Watchers. These are some of the most common weight loss diets known to all Americans. What happens if they fail? Some people have turned to a radical, yet very successful surgery in order to lose weight. The procedure, laparoscopic Roux-en-Y gastric bypass, has been performed since the mid-1990s with dramatic results.

WHAT IS WEIGHT LOSS SURGERY? Weight loss surgery, also called bariatric surgery, is a corrective surgical procedure that effectively allows a person to lose weight. This surgery is the last resort for patients who have not been able to lose weight by traditional means. Morbid obesity is usually defined in males as 100 pounds over ideal weight and 80 pounds in females. There is also a body mass index (BMI) over 40.

In order to qualify for the surgery, patients must exhibit other medical problems caused by obesity such as diabetes, arthritis, sleep apnea, heart disease, high blood pressure or high cholesterol. The risks of the co-morbidities must outweigh the risks of the surgery.

WHAT ARE THE TYPES OF SURGERY? There are two categories of weight loss surgery, which include restrictive surgery and malabsorptive surgery.

Restrictive surgery promotes weight loss by making a portion of the stomach smaller, which ultimately restricts the amount of food held by the stomach. This does not interfere with the process of digestion. Two types of surgeries performed include adjustable gastric banding and vertical banded gastroplasty. Both procedures make the stomach into a small pouch, only allowing for a minimal amount of food to be taken into the stomach.

Malabsorptive procedures have become most common and they involve restricting stomach size and bypassing a portion of the small intestine. A bypass of the small intestine is made directly from the stomach to the small intestine, which prevents absorption of calories and nutrients.

WHAT IS THE ROUX-EN-Y GASTRIC BYPASS? This procedure is the most common with excellent success and minimal complications. The stomach is made into a small pouch, that allows for a small amount of food intake. Next, a Y-shaped section of the small intestine is attached to the pouch, bypassing a majority of the stomach and the first portion of the small intestine. Ultimately, the body can only take in a small amount of food and there is minimal absorption. This process allows for weight loss.

IS THIS SUCCESSFUL? This surgery is very successful, with almost all patients losing up to 100 pounds. In addition, many of the other related medical problems resolve with the weight loss. For example, over 90 percent of patients with non-insulin dependent diabetes resolved their condition and did not require medication to control their blood sugar. Over 85 percent of all patients with high blood pressure were able to get their blood pressure under control. Other studies have shown patients were able to reduce their cholesterol, resolve sleep apnea and the pains of arthritis disappeared.

WHAT ARE THE COMPLICATIONS? Wound infections are the most common postoperative surgical problem encountered after weight loss surgery. Other surgical complications have included a leak in the surgical site, internal infection, blood clot in the legs or lung, gallbladder disease and bowel obstruction. Overall, the surgery has been perfected and it is performed through the laparoscope, allowing for small incisions, less infections and a faster recovery.

IS THIS COSTLY? In general, the cost is about $15,000 and many health insurances are covering the procedure when it is deemed medically necessary. If a person is considering this surgery, a conference with your doctor and insurance provider will probably be required

WHAT SHOULD I DO? If you are morbidly obese and conventional diets have failed, you may want to consider this surgery, especially if you have other medical problems. You will need to discuss this with your primary health care provider. Then, you will need to be referred to an experienced surgeon in bariatric surgery. You will want to ask the doctor about the procedures available, number performed, complication rate and success rate. This is a very radical way to lose weight, but it may be a method to providing a fulfilling and healthy lifestyle.

ectopic pregnancy

Early pregnancy with abdominal pain can signal a problem and needs timely evaluation. In the United States, about one to two percent of all pregnancies occur outside the uterus and are called an ectopic pregnancy. This is a serious health issue for the woman and medical attention must be sought from a health care provider.

WHAT IS AN ECTOPIC PREGNANCY? An ectopic pregnancy is where a fertilized ovum implants itself outside the woman's uterus. The implanted fertile egg is usually found in the fallopian tube. The fallopian tube is the tube that connects the ovary and the uterus, and carries the egg during the normal reproductive cycle down from the ovary to the uterus.

An ectopic pregnancy is sometimes called a tubal pregnancy, abdominal pregnancy or cervical pregnancy. The implantation usually occurs within the fallopian tube, but it can occur in the ovary, abdominal cavity or in the cervix.

WHAT ARE THE SYMPTOMS? Ectopic pregnancies are usually diagnosed within the first two months of pregnancy. A couple of situations may exist whereby a woman is diagnosed with an ectopic pregnancy. In the first situation right-or left-sided pain may develop as the pregnancy progresses and the tubal pregnancy is incidentally diagnosed due to pain. The pain is usually located in the right or left lower quadrant of the abdomen between the ovaries and bladder.

The other situation that exists is when a woman may not realize that she is pregnant and then suddenly develops very severe pain, weakness, abnormal vaginal bleeding, and low blood pressure. This usually signals that the ectopic pregnancy has ruptured and the woman is bleeding internally. This is a surgical emergency and the woman needs to be immediately evaluated by her health care provider. This is a serious and life-threatening condition.

It is important to remember that the symptoms may range from mild to severe including a missed period, cramping, vaginal bleeding, hemorrhage, and shock. Health care providers must always be suspect of pregnancy in females with functioning ovaries.

WHY DOES THIS OCCUR? The risks for tubal pregnancy are many and the greatest risk is having previously had an ectopic pregnancy. Other risk factors include damage to the fallopian tube by trauma, a previous sexually transmitted disease like Chlamydia, congenital abnormalities of the tubes, tumors or use of birth control methods such as intrauterine devices (IUD). It is important to consult with your doctor if you possess any of these risks prior to pregnancy.

HOW IS THIS DIAGNOSED? A health care provider must always be suspect in pregnant women that present with complaints of abdominal pain. Pregnancy must be diagnosed and another blood test may be used to follow the levels of the hormone of pregnancy, called the human chorionic gonadotropin (HCG). Pelvic exam may reveal tenderness in the area of either fallopian tube. Finally, an ultrasound of the pelvis may show the enlarging mass in the tube. If there is bleeding and rupture, this will also be seen on ultrasound. Sometimes surgery is necessary to make a diagnosis.

WHAT IS THE TREATMENT? Once diagnosis is made, removal of the tubal pregnancy is necessary. If caught early, medicines can be used to induce the passage of the fertilized ovum. This is not too common.

Most commonly, a woman will require surgery to remove the ectopic pregnancy. This may be done through a laparoscope or through an open surgical procedure. If diagnosed in the earlier stages prior to rupture and hemorrhage, the fallopian tube can be opened and repaired. If diagnosis is delayed and rupture occurs, the tube may be permanently damaged and may need to be removed. Delayed diagnosis can result in death of the woman.

WHAT ELSE SHOULD BE DONE? Prevention of an ectopic pregnancy is essential through the practice of safe sexual habits and avoiding sexually transmitted diseases. If you are not at risk and are experiencing pain and bleeding with pregnancy, you must be medically evaluated. Pay attention to your body. If you have previously had an ectopic pregnancy, you are at risk again, but, 85 percent of these women are able to achieve a normal pregnancy free of complications. Be sure to seek medical attention if you have concerns.

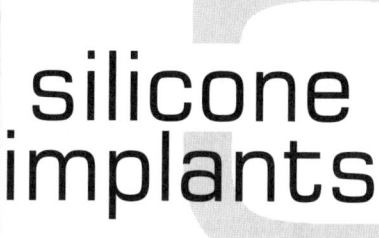

silicone implants

An advisory panel completed an evaluation on the use of silicone breast implants and votes 9-6 in favor for reinstating their use. This ruling reverses an 11-year ban on the use of silicone breast implants in the United States. Only saline implants have been available to women for surgical augmentation since 1992.

WHAT ARE IMPLANTS? In the early 1960s, two plastic surgeons developed the concept of silicone breast implants. The implant was initially manufactured by Dow Corning in New York. The intent was for plastic surgical correction of female breast deformity after breast cancer surgery. In addition, the implants were used for augmentation for cosmetic enhancement. For nearly 30 years, silicone implants were used successfully and without difficulty.

WHAT ARE THE COMPLICATIONS? Over the years, female patients began to develop some complications after the use of the silicone implants. The biggest problem was implant leak or rupture. The failure rate of the implant after about 15 years was nearly 25 percent. This is true of all breast implants, saline or silicone.

It was thought that the leaking silicone contributed to systemic medical conditions such as increased risks of cancer. It was also thought that there was an increased risk of connective tissue disorders such as rheumatoid arthritis and fibromyalgia. Silicone implants were also thought to interfere with reproduction and the ability to breast-feed., and that women with implants had a higher risk of suicide.

WHAT HAPPENED? After a variety of these concerns and complications were raised, public outcry resulted in the FDA banning the production and use of silicone implants in 1992. The replacement implant developed was made of saline. Silicone is a manufactured substance that is in gel form.

Several medical devices such as heart valve coatings and intravenous catheters are made of silicone. The body does not usually react to its presence. Saline is salt water and was thought to be safer. Cosmetically, it is thought that the silicone implants provided a much more natural appearance than the saline implants. Therefore, several research organizations studied the claims regarding silicone implants.

WHAT RESEARCH OCCURRED? The Mayo Clinic, Harvard Medical School, and the Academy of Sciences have studied this issue. Plastic Surgeons felt that patients needed a choice in implants and this provided the impetus for the studies.

Research has concluded that silicone implants leak and rupture at the same rate as saline implants. Due to the presence of the silicone gel, the leak is slower than saline implants. There was no increased risk for cancer amongst women with silicone implants. Mammography is not less sensitive in women with silicone implants. The incidence of connective tissue disorders is not any higher in women with these implants, nor is breast-feeding affected. Also, suicide rates and death rates are not higher in these individuals, compared to peers in similar situations.

WHAT ARE THE RISKS OF IMPLANTS? Whether silicone or saline implants are used, the severe risks are the same. Infection in the breast that results in the removal of the implant leads to cosmetic deformity. Additionally, an aggressive infection can severely damage the appearance and shape of the breast. The risk of leakage and rupture increases with time and additional surgery and replacement may be necessary. Overall, the chances of life-threatening illnesses are not greater with silicone versus saline implants according to medical research.

WHAT SHOULD YOU DO? In the event that you need cosmetic breast surgery after cancer or simple cosmetic augmentation, seek out a board-certified plastic surgeon with vast experience. Be sure to complete appropriate research and be an informed consumer prior to surgical intervention.

death with dignity

A majority of my articles focus on a specific medical problem, including the pathophysiology, disease process, signs, symptoms and treatment. This is because I practice evidence-based medicine--which means that what I do on a daily basis is founded on medical literature and current recommended practice guidelines.

Those guidelines are constantly evolving with advances in science. The treatment I may have recommended six months ago, can be different from what I would advise today. Thus, keeping abreast of the science of medical practice is important in providing the best possible care. But, emotion and empathy are just as important. It is my hope that I am able to provide emotional support during a time of crisis that parallels the quality of my medical care.

Recently, I was involved in a case that has had a tremendous emotional impact on me and my staff. In nearly 20 years of practice, I have not experienced such a situation. Let me share some of the details.

An elderly gentleman presented to the emergency department with complaints of jaw, neck, shoulder and chest pain. His pain came on in the middle of the night and was the worst that he had ever experienced. It seemed to wax and wane, so he decided to come in during my morning shift. He was not really interested in giving me a history, but wanted me to treat his pain. Because he admitted that he did not often seek medical care, the fact that this tough, old guy wanted me to treat his pain indicated how severe it was.

This presentation was clearly an emergency and a CT scan of the chest was necessary. We needed to act fast because I was concerned that this was a classic presentation of a dissecting thoracic aortic aneurysm—a life-threatening condition in which a weakened wall of the aorta can bulge or balloon, then rupture and cause internal bleeding. I provided pain relief after my exam and whisked him off to the CT scanner.

In a few minutes, my worst fears were confirmed by a frantic call from the radiologist reading the CT scan. This pleasant gentleman, with a dry sense of humor, had an aneurysm that started in his heart and extended to his kidneys. One kidney was already affected by the growing aneurysm. Blood flow was being impaired and immediate cardiothoracic surgery was necessary. In addition, the CT scan revealed a new lung cancer.

After I presented this case to the patient and his family, he told me that he was a widower who missed his wife. He stated that despite his family, he was very lonely. In addition, he had chronic arthritic pains and back pain--he could no longer do the activities that he loved. The medical information that I provided to him was very grim, and he stated that it was his time. He wanted to be with his wife and felt that he had had a good life. Quality of life was important to him and now his was poor.

I outlined the risks, benefits and alternatives of his conditions. Without surgery, his chance of survival was less than 10 percent. Even with surgery, he had a 40 percent chance of dying. If he did survive, he would face radiation and chemotherapy for his lung cancer. This dear man let me know that he wanted to die with dignity and in comfort. He saw his wife suffer with cancer and he did not want to go through this ordeal.

As a physician I have a duty to preserve life, but I must respect the wishes of my patients. There is nothing wrong with not undertaking extraordinary means to preserve life. This was clearly a terminal situation and I wanted to make my new friend happy and comfortable. He asked for a phone after his family had left and he contacted a funeral home to make his own arrangements. After that was done, he asked to return home to die.

His final request was that I keep him comfortable, as he did not want to experience the extreme pain of his condition. I provided the strongest pain medication available and he left, thanking me for my care and compassion. He died that evening in the company of his family.

A few days later, a nurse told me that as he left, he wanted everyone to know that he could not thank them enough for respecting his wishes, being honest about his condition, and allowing him to die with dignity.

This is what medicine is truly about and I will never forget him.

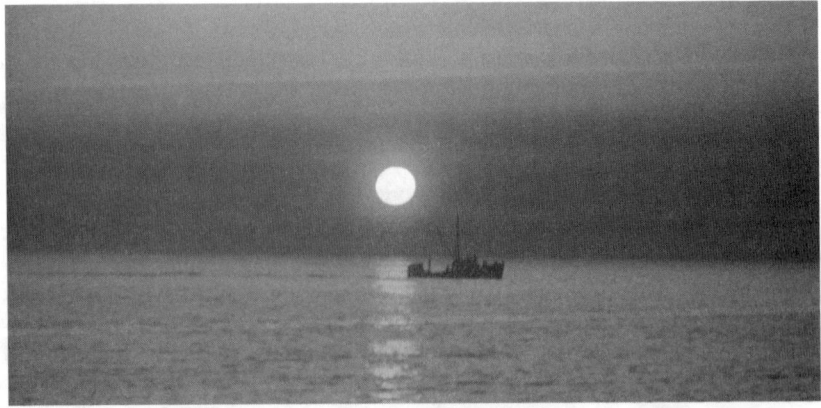

To Your Health with Dr. Wojo